Therapy as Learning

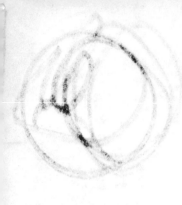

". . . but whatever we learn has a purpose and whatever we do affects everything and everyone else, if even only in the tiniest way. . . . And it's much the same thing with knowledge, for whenever you learn something new, the whole world is that much richer."

NORTON JUSTIN
The Phantom Tollbooth

*"I'd rather learn
from one small bird
how to sing than
teach ten thousand stars
how not to dance"*

e e cummings

Therapy as Learning

RICHARD K. SCHWARTZ, M.S., O.T.R.

Associate Professor of Occupational Therapy
Associate Professor of Physical Medicine and Rehabilitation
The University of Texas Health Science Center
at San Antonio, TX.

With the assistance of
DAVID E. COCHRANE, Ph.D.,
Associate Professor of Biology, Tufts University, Medford, MA, on
Chapter 1.

Illustrated by
JUNE CHAMBERLAIN, B.S.,
Department of Biology, Tufts University, Medford, MA.

THE AMERICAN OCCUPATIONAL THERAPY

ASSOCIATION, INC.

Rockville, Maryland

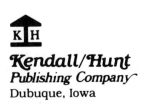

Kendall/Hunt
Publishing Company
Dubuque, Iowa

For Gayle S. Fish, B.S.,O.T.R.

My student, my wife, my teacher, my friend.

Copyright © 1985 by The American Occupational Therapy Association

Library of Congress Catalog Card Number: 85–50743

ISBN 0–8403–3595–4

Printed in the United States of America
B   403595   01

Contents

1/16/87

Catalog

v

Acknowledgments

Many people assisted in the preparation of this manuscript, and I am grateful to them all. I am especially indebted to the following:

Martha Kirkland, Alice Bowker, Virginia Scardina, Dottie Wilson, and Gretchen Reeves who, along with the Special Interest Sections in Physical Disabilities and Sensory Integration of the American Occupational Therapy Association, sponsored this monograph;

David E. Cochrane, Ph.D., of Tufts University for teaching me cellular neurobiology both in his classroom and first-hand in his laboratory, and June Chamberlain, also of Tufts University, for her excellent illustrations;

John P. Scholz, M.A., L.P.T., formerly Assistant Professor of Physical Therapy at the University of Texas Health Science Center at San Antonio and presently a doctoral student in the Department of Experimental Psychology at the University of Connecticut, Storrs, CT, and Janet L. Dubinsky, Ph.D., Department of Anatomy and Neurobiology, Washington University School of Medicine, St. Louis, MO, for their critical comments on this manuscript during the revision process;

Gene Constantine, Victoria Gonzales, Andrea Sherman, and Tracy Ferlet, all student-therapists, who assisted me at various times;

Lisa Haby, Lucy Kilmer, and especially Jaqueline Caver for their assistance in the preparation and typing of the manuscript;

Dr. F. G. Antonson, my former Program Director, and Dr. Charles H. Christiansen, my present Program Director, for their support of my efforts;

My sister, Jane Schwartz, whose own struggles to write her first novel gave her a special viewpoint on writing that inspired me to continue in spite of the difficulties inherent in writing a book;

My son Benjamin for persisting at coming in to see me and play with me while I was writing;

And most especially, to my wife Gayle who wants me to spend my life doing the things which make me happy and who has helped me immeasurably with every phase of research and writing.

Introduction

All animals have adaptively evolved in numerous and varied ways to benefit from their experiences and interactions with the world. The nervous system has been called, ". . . Nature's greatest invention for enabling organisms to deal competently with their environment." (Granit, 1977). One of the most obvious and yet mysterious ways in which nervous systems serve adaptation of the individual is called learning. But what is learning?

Learning is the process whereby an individual modifies responsiveness to stimuli or acquires new patterns of behavior as a result of previous interactions with the environment, not including those changes due to growth, maturation, or aging, those caused by disease or trauma, or those that reflect a change in levels of awareness or motivation (although one can *learn* to become more aware and/or more motivated). Learning only occurs when changes in behavior outlast the stimuli that cause such changes.

In 1978, the Eleanor Clarke Slagle Lecture was presented by Lorna Jean King at the Annual Conference of the American Occupational Therapy Association. Her address was titled, "Toward a Science of Adaptive Response." Two admonitions that bear repeating were given in the preface to her remarks. First, "To allow future specialization [within the profession] to result in further fragmentation, might well be suicidal. Therefore, *we need a framework that will give specialists the bond of a common structure* (emphasis added)." Second, "We may develop complex theories, but to be really useful, they will need to be based on a straightforward structure that can be easily understood and that is clearly related to the client's life functions."

These are the aims of this monograph: First, to provide a common framework for all clinicians regardless of discipline or specialization. Second, to present a straightforward structure that patients and therapists alike may appreciate. Learning concepts provide an especially appropriate framework for the analysis of therapeutic activities. They

ix

focus attention not only on events that occur at the cellular level, but also on events that occur at the level of social interactions. The learning process transcends the specific concerns of specializations within therapy professions. One further advantage of this perspective is that almost everyone, from layperson to professional, child to adult, has some familiarity with the activities and processes of learning. Although the term "therapist" is used frequently, it is appropriate to substitute the terms "clinician," "educator," "nurse," or any other referring to the role of assisting patients to change their behaviors.

An individual's retention of behavioral changes is generally considered to be a function of memory. Any separation of the concept of learning from that of memory is an artificial distinction with respect to adaptive processes. If changes in competence or independence of the individual cannot be stored and retrieved, the process of therapy cannot be very effective. Memory, in its broadest sense, as opposed to simply the conscious recall of information, does not separate those mechanisms which modify behavior (learning) from those that sustain such modifications (memory). It is beyond the scope of this monograph to explore memory per se. Only the *longevity* and *retention* of the various types of learning will be considered. Issues of retention will be explored in relation to the planning and sequencing of intervention activities.

Changes in behavior, which occur due to growth and development, aging, trauma, and illness, are also important parts of the adaptive process. Although there is no specific term for such changes, they all fall into a broader class of events (as does learning). This more general adaptive process is termed "plasticity." It refers to changes within neural systems which result in prolonged alterations of cellular and/ or synaptic function that, in principle, could account for behavioral modification (Kandel 1976; Buchtel and Berlucci 1977).

The role of a clinician or therapist is to alter pathologic or dysfunctional response patterns and to increase independent, goal-directed activity. To do this, practitioners must know which treatment methods can predictably improve performance beyond the level permitted by natural recovery processes. Intervention must speed the rate of recovery, or slow the rate of decline, or increase the degree of function above that which would occur without treatment.

Many therapists perceive correctly that a major part of their role is to teach, direct, and guide patients toward functional improvement. It is generally assumed that therapists teach their patients and that these patients are capable of learning. Many therapists are familiar with the rules of learning and reinforcement, yet neglect to take the time to consciously and carefully analyze therapeutic intervention with respect to learning. It is rare that therapists observe the principles of learning in any rigorous or controlled manner. This is unfortunate because the greater the ability of a teacher to monitor and control the stimuli reaching a learner, the better the learning results will be.

Teachers are not essential for learning. For example, if you eat a new food and it makes you sick, you will very likely avoid that food in the future. Learning has occurred through rapid aversive conditioning, without the intervention of an "instructor." Learning occurs when certain patterns of temporal and spatial stimulation are registered within a nervous system and bring about behavioral changes that outlast these events.

Teachers or therapists must ensure that the required stimulation occurs and that the learner is capable of responding. Consistency in providing experiences for patients will induce desired changes in behavior, and thus ensure teaching success. Therapists must select and direct the experiences (and therefore the environmental stimulation) of their clients in ways that will change behaviors from maladaptive to adaptive. If therapists could better analyze the sensations and motor responses associated with particular behaviors and determine the patterns of neural activity associated with such performance, it is plausible that they might be able to better modify the patterns of neural activity of a patient's nervous system.

An exciting recent discovery by neurobiologists is the principle that temporal and spatial *patterning of synaptic activity* in neural circuits occurring as a result of environmental stimulation determines whether learning will occur. Even more remarkable is that the *patterning of stimuli* determines whether learning will be of short-term, intermediate, or long-term duration. The elucidation of these principles over the past few years by Kandel (1976, 1979a, 1979b, 1981) and others requires that therapists revise and expand their awareness of the role of learning in relation to patient treatments.

Recent research in cellular neurobiology, applied physiology, and human neurosciences, provide therapists with information that will be most useful in developing more rational and scientific methods of treating various neurological and learning disabilities. Unfortunately, advances in basic science are often difficult to translate into therapeutic actions without a framework in which the clinical significance of these "facts" can be organized, interpreted, and ultimately evaluated. A further difficulty has been the problem of being able to appropriately generalize the results of studies performed using nonhuman animals to clinical intervention with humans. These problems complicate the process of being able to translate basic neurobiological research to the study of human learning. There are, however, general principles that appear to be valid across species. Certain of these principles have already been tested to determine if they apply equally well to humans as to lower phyla; others remain as yet untested using human subjects.

Of course, for therapists to teach it is assumed that patients are capable of learning. Therapy should be viewed as a learning process. Therapists therefore need basic information on the neural events associated with different kinds of learning and the conditions under which the opportunities for learning are greatest. Basic principles of nervous systems and types of learning will be described. Current therapeutic practices will be analyzed according to these principles. Finally, the implications of learning and neuroscience theories for future research into the theoretical foundations of treatment principles will be suggested and discussed.

This monograph has both heuristic and practical implications for the conduct of therapy. Its aim is to provide clinicians with information that will increase the precision with which they select activities, and thus maximize both the rate and extent of learning. If therapists are more knowledgeable concerning the neural events associated with treatment and the patterns of neural activity associated with learning, it follows that this knowledge will be used and will lead to therapeutic learning. Total precision in the use of therapeutic activity to scientifically elicit adaptive responses is a remote and perhaps unattainable goal. What is increasingly possible in light of developments in basic science research is that therapists can greatly *improve* their effectiveness in the choice and application of activity designed to modify client performance. This monograph will serve as a reminder that any attempt to apply these ideas to patient treatment must remain experimental.

The degree to which therapists can monitor and control environmental information impacts on their ability to assist patients to learn and/or relearn control of their own bodies. Therapists are vitally interested in analyzing and understanding events that take place within the patients' nervous systems, but even under ideal circumstances they have only indirect access to such events. Therapists are concerned with understanding the neurophysiologic and neurodevelopmental bases of behaviors they observe. To do this, it is necessary to draw upon the knowledge of many disciplines including the medical sciences, biology, psychology, and education.

To *teach* patients to control movements and perceptions, it is imperative that one understand motoric and perceptual *learning*. What changes occur within patients when they practice an activity? How long can these changes, seen in a single session of treatment, endure? What are the necessary conditions for the nervous system to learn and to retain control of voluntary functions? To answer these questions one must understand and recognize changes that occur at the neural level during learning. Although therapists may not conduct such investigations, they must be knowledgeable about basic neurosciences and ensure that basic research addresses questions and problems that they confront daily in the clinical setting.

Principles of Nervous Systems

with DAVID E. COCHRANE, Ph.D.

Neuroscience can provide therapists with a more detailed and clearer understanding of both normal and pathologic conditions. Many of these conditions are complex yet essential for the understanding of human behavior. Inasmuch as learning requires practice, readers may find it necessary to reread this material more than once.

HUMAN NERVOUS SYSTEM CONCEPTS AND TERMINOLOGY

If the fifty billion individual neurons of the human nervous system were randomly arranged, without order or logic to their interconnections, the result would be chaos. But such is not the case; neurons are grouped by location and/or function. During the past 5 years, neurotransmitter research has shown that neurons do not need proximity to be organized into a functional unit. Although neurons themselves are remarkably similar, groupings into specialized functional units have evolved so that each region of the nervous system is both anatomically and functionally distinct.

Many neuroscientists have arbitrarily chosen to describe the nervous system as being organized into three major functional divisions: the central nervous system, the autonomic nervous system, and the peripheral somatic nervous system. The central nervous system regulates and coordinates activity throughout the body. It includes the brain, brain stem, and spinal cord. The autonomic nervous system serves to ensure the survival of the individual by maintaining the internal environment of the body within the narrow boundaries compatible with life; that is homeostasis. The autonomic nervous system is further subdivided into sympathetic and parasympathetic divisions. The sympathetic division governs our responses to stress and emergency situations. The parasympathetic division maintains vegetative functions of the body and restores the body to normal after stress or emergencies. Under most conditions, the balance between sympathetic and parasympathetic activity maintains the constancy of our internal environment. The somatic (peripheral) nervous system consists of peripheral nerves. These transmit sensory information about the body and the external environment into the central nervous system along afferent neurons. They also carry motor commands from the central nervous system to effector organs along efferent neuronal pathways.

Functional groupings of neuron cell bodies are a distinct feature of nervous system organization. Where such groupings are found in the central nervous system (CNS), they are termed *nuclei*. Similar groupings outside the CNS (within the autonomic or somatic nervous system) are termed *ganglia*. The existence of nuclei and ganglia establishes boundary conditions on the interconnections that are possible among neurons. Relationships between groups of nerve cells are represented by *tracts* or pathways which connect such structures to one another. Tracts enable communication between structural units of the nervous system. A tract may be efferent, afferent, or associational with respect to the information it conveys. Familiar examples of efferent tracts include corticospinal, rubrospinal, reticulospinal, and vestibulospinal pathways. Examples of afferent tracts include the dorsal column/medial lemniscal, spinothalamic, and trigeminothalamic pathways. Associational tracts include the corpus callosum and the pathways of the anterior and posterior commissures. The bulk of the "white" matter of the nervous system is composed of myelinated axons of these functional tracts.

It is impossible to describe the action of every neuron in the nervous system. To understand how neurons regulate and control behavior of the whole organism, it is necessary to focus on smaller functional units. These may contain only a few neurons or up to several million neurons. One of the simplest functional units of the human nervous system is the myotatic stretch reflex (Fig. 1), which helps to maintain the length of a muscle against sudden or unexpected loads, among other things. If we sharply tap the tendon of a muscle, such as the quadriceps femoris, the fibers of the muscle and of the muscle spindle are lengthened. The stretch reflex simply and quickly restores the initial length of the muscle by causing it to contract.

This reflex is often described as requiring only two neurons to achieve its purpose. It is a highly localized reflex resulting in excitation of the muscle whose fibers (and stretch receptor organs) are lengthened. The primary muscle spindle (IA) afferents also provide collateral inputs to interneurons which inhibit excitation of antagonistic motor neurons. These actions are often considered the "stretch reflex" (Carew 1981). Embedded within the muscle and arranged in parallel with its fibers is the muscle spindle, a stretch receptor organ

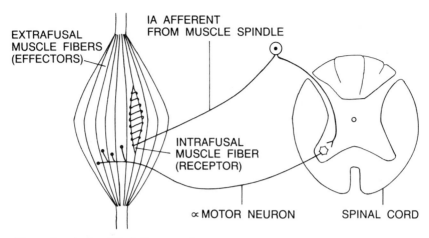

Figure 1.   A simplified diagram of a myotatic stretch reflex.

that sends sensory (IA afferent) fibers to the spinal cord. When the muscle spindle is stretched, the low threshold IA afferent fibers convey a series of action potentials monosynaptically to the alpha motor neurons of that muscle. The influence of the IA afferents is such that they cause the alpha motor neurons to fire a train of action potentials to the muscle of origin. This efferent discharge causes the muscle to contract and thus acts to restore the original resting length of the muscle (Brodal 1981; Noback and Demarest 1975). All therapists should be familiar with this reflex arc. Perhaps not so obvious is that this organizational unit is an oversimplified abstraction. It is *not* the two neuron pathways from muscle spindle back to the muscle that are oversimplified. Oversimplification arises because, at any given moment, each motor neuron receives inputs not only from IA spindle afferents but from a multitude of other spinal segmental and supraspinal sources. Descriptions of nervous system organization (such as the stretch reflex) are meaningful not because they present a true picture of the interconnectivity of neurons, but because they permit functionally accurate descriptions of events too complex to represent in their entirety. *All* descriptions of functional units of the human nervous system are actually conceptual abstractions. Even complex descriptions of stretch reflexes (Scholz and Campbell 1980) are "simplified" views of actual neural events. Whether the focus is a simple reflex arc or complex events serving learning, it is not possible to present the "true" and "complete" picture of the interconnections of all neurons participating in a given behavior.

Focusing on an alpha motor neuron (αMN) a simplified functional diagram can be used to illustrate certain major sources of input (Fig. 2). The alpha motor neuron (Final Common Pathway) and all muscle

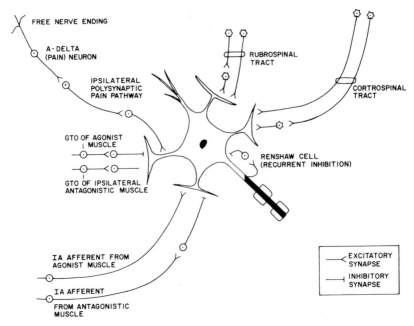

Figure 2.   A schematic representation of some of the important synaptic inputs to an alpha motor neuron.

fibers innervated by this neuron are collectively referred to as the "Motor Unit." A typical motor neuron receives input from approximately 10,000 synapses. Clearly it is not possible to diagram and label each input! Figure 2, therefore, is a simplified representation of some of the important sources of inputs and the nature of their primary effect on the motor neuron, be it inhibitory or excitatory. Just as it is not possible to diagram and label each input to a motor neuron, it is not usually possible to diagram those muscle fibers that are served by even a single motor neuron. Although certain muscles responsible for finely controlled movements may have motor units with only 5 to 10 muscle cells innervated by its motor neuron, most muscles have motor unit ratios (the number of muscle fibers served by a single motor neuron) from 50 to 1500! Even though total and complete descriptions of neural events serving human behavior are impossible, it is possible to grasp much of what occurs in our nervous system by understanding the physiologic and anatomic *principles* that determine the behavior of individual neurons and their interactions with one another. It is our experience that most students wishing to appreciate the neurobiological bases of learning first need to review the principles and mechanisms that follow.

MORPHOLOGICAL AND ULTRASTRUCTURAL CHARACTERISTICS OF NEURONS

The fundamental unit of the nervous system is the individual nerve cell or *neuron*. The cell body of a neuron has the genetic material and metabolic machinery common to all cells. Yet, unlike most other cells, neurons do not divide after birth; we are born with all the neurons we will ever have. Neurons represent approximately one-tenth of the total number of cells of the nervous system. The remaining nine-tenths are *glial cells* which serve to nourish the neurons, to regulate the ionic concentration of the extracellular fluid space, and to physically support the neurons. One type of glial cell, termed astroglia, also serves an important phagocytotic function for removing the remains of damaged neurons. Astroglial proliferation following injury to the CNS can lead to "plaque" or scar formation and result in nervous system malfunction (Barr and Kiernan 1983). Glial cells are generally much smaller than neurons, so that neurons account for some 50% of the total cell volume.

Neurons come in a variety of sizes and shapes, but generally can be divided into three functional classes: efferent neurons, afferent neurons, and interneurons. Efferent neurons carry information from the central nervous system (CNS) to the various effector cells. An example already cited is the αMN that innervates skeletal muscle. Afferent neurons carry information into the CNS. At their endings in the periphery are receptors, which respond to a variety of physical and/or chemical changes in the internal or external environment by producing nerve impulses. Interneurons, which account for 99% of all nerve cells, lie entirely within the CNS and carry information between CNS neurons. The number of interneurons between afferent and efferent neurons varies from none (as in circuitry of the stretch reflex) to many thousands or millions as in such complex processes as visual perception. All neurons—afferent, efferent, and interneurons—have unique features that distinguish them from other cells. These include a distinct shape, a cell membrane that can generate nerve impulses, and the synapse, a structure for transferring information from the neuron to an effector cell or other neuron. In addition to these features, all neurons have common parts, including dendrites, cell body, axon, and the nerve terminals. The *dendrites* are a series of branched projections from the cell body and are generally involved in carrying information to the cell body. Their membranes have regions that specialize in recognizing and responding to specific neurotransmitters. The *cell body* contains the nucleus, mitochondria, rough endoplasmic reticulum, Golgi apparatus, and other cellular organelles necessary for cell metabolism, synthesis, growth, and repair. The cell body is responsible for nourishing the entire neuron. The *axon* or nerve fiber (not to be confused with what is commonly called a nerve, which is a bundle of nerve fibers) is a single process extending from the cell body and is generally associated with carrying information away from the cell body. Axons are often long, sometimes more than a meter, as in spinal motor neurons, but may also be short, as in local circuit association-type neurons or interneurons. The first portion of the axon, as it leaves the cell body, is called the initial segment, and here the action potential arises in response to neurotransmitter action at the specialized regions of the dendrites. The action of neurotransmitter at the dendrites causes a change in membrane potential, which spreads to the initial segment as a result of the passive electrical properties of the dendritic and cell body membranes. The action potential is generated first at the initial segment because the membrane of this segment has a lower threshold of excitability (i.e., closer to the resting membrane potential) than the membrane of the intervening cell body. This will be explained later in this chapter.

Axons often branch and give off right-angled collateral axonal processes and, near their ends, branch considerably to end as *terminals*. The nerve terminal is responsible for releasing the chemical transmitter substance that will affect the postsynaptic membrane of the next neuron or effector cell, such as muscle. Mammalian peripheral nerve axons are surrounded by a fatty sheath known as *myelin*. This sheath is interrupted at regular intervals of a millimeter or less by *nodes of Ranvier*. Myelin is formed from many closely packed layers of Schwann cell membranes; consequently, there is no communication between the axon and the extracellular fluid, except where the myelin and axon are surrounded by connective tissue sheath, the endoneurium. Because of its fatty nature, myelin acts as an insulator and, therefore, has considerable effect on the electrical properties of the nerve fiber.

In the central nervous system, myelin sheathing is formed by glial cells called oligodendroglia. These cells are one principal type of neurologia; a second type is astrocytes. Astrocytes are generally thought to function as insulators and to provide an important component of the blood/brain barrier (Barr and Kiernan 1983). They are commonly found in regions of axons, dendrites, and along capillary walls within the CNS. The site of communication between the axon of a neuron and another neuron or effector cell is called a *synapse*. Chemical synapses—those that involve the release of specific transmitter substances—are of five basic types: the neuromuscular junction (the synapse between a motor neuron and muscle cell), the axodendritic synapse (between the axonal terminal of one neuron and the dendritic membrane of another), the axosomatic synapse, formed when an axonal terminal synapses with the cell body of another neuron, dendrodendritic synapses, between two dendrites of adjacent neurons and axo-axonal synapses between two axons of adjacent neurons. The latter two were considered rare until recently but have been reported in many parts of the nervous system, and are generally inhibitory. All synapses have three basic components: (1) a presynaptic nerve terminal—that specialized ending of the neuron which contains synaptic vesicles (a subcellular organelle that usually contains neurotransmitter) and the machinery for releasing transmitter; (2) a synaptic cleft, an interstitial space of 10–20 nm which separates the nerve terminal from the postsynaptic membrane; and (3) a postsynaptic cell with a specialized membrane immediately opposite the nerve terminal. Several substances are known to be neurotransmitters (Cooper et al. 1978) and many more chemicals are suspected of being neurotransmitters (putative transmitters). Each neuron may contain one or more of these neurotransmitters. Another class of chemicals found in the CNS, called neuromodulators, are responsible for modifying the action of neurotransmitters.

MEMBRANES

Neurons, like other cells, are dependent on membranes to maintain their integrity and to provide selective barriers that maintain the internal cell environment essential for normal cell function. For example, the plasma membrane separates the aqueous intracellular fluid, with its higher concentration of potassium, from the extracellular fluid environment having a higher sodium concentration. Membranes are well suited for this function because they are composed primarily of lipids and protein and thus can readily form interfaces between two such aqueous environments. The lipids of cell membranes are of three kinds: neutral fats, phospholipids, and cholesterol. Of these, phospholipids are by far the most numerous and form the bilayer backbone of the cell membrane. Phospholipids have a distinct polar or lipophobic ("lipid-hating") group at one end and a long, nonpolar or lipophilic ("lipid-loving") tail at the other. Thus, they arrange themselves into a bilayer interface with their lipophobic groups facing out toward the intracellular and extracellular aqueous environments and their lipophilic tails pointing inward, thereby forming a nonpolar interior (Fig. 3). This phospholipid bilayer is not a rigid, static structure, but fluid and capable of change. The proteins of cell membranes are embedded in this lipid bilayer and, because of the fluid nature of the bilayer, are themselves mobile. This dynamic model of cell membranes was originally proposed by Singer and Nicolson (1972) and is called the "fluid-mosaic model." Today, it is the most widely accepted model of cell membranes.

Carbohydrates are the third class of molecules found in cell mem-

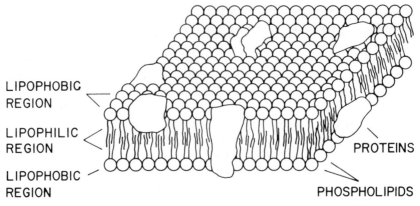

LIPOPHOBIC
REGION

LIPOPHILIC
REGION

LIPOPHOBIC
REGION

PROTEINS

PHOSPHOLIPIDS

Figure 3.   The nerve cell membrane in accord with the "fluid mosaic" model
of Singer and Nicolson (1972).

branes. They are present in a very low percentage and are usually
associated with proteins. The carbohydrates of cell membranes play a
very important role in the recognition of particular molecules in the
extracellular environment.

THE BASIS OF NEURONAL EXCITABILITY

Bioelectricity and the Passive Properties of Cell Membranes

Electric charge is a fundamental property of matter and the basic unit
of electrical measurement. There are two types of charge: positive ($+$)
and negative ($-$) and they behave symmetrically. It is a fundamental
law of nature that like charges (e.g., two positives) repel each other,
and that unlike charges (i.e., negative and positive) attract each other.
This attraction between *unlike* charges can be measured and the factors that affect the amount of attraction studied. For example, the
force of attraction between unlike charges is a function of the quantity
of charge and the distance separating them. The amount of this force
increases as the two unlike charges move closer together and it also
increases as the quantity of charge gets larger.

   To separate unlike charges, that is, to move a positive and negative
charge apart, external force must be applied. Energy is therefore
added to the system, and we perform work (W) which in physics is
defined as a force (F) moved over some distance (X); $W = FX$. If the
separated unlike charges are allowed to move together, *they* will do
work because they will be exerting a force over some distance. Thus,
when unlike electric charges are separated by some distance, they
have the *potential* to do work. This potential is called *voltage*. Voltage is
a measure of the potential of separated electric charges to do work,

the amount of work that is done by an electric charge when it moves from one point in a system to another point. Voltage is also called electromotive force (EMF) and is always measured between two points. We express the measurement of voltage in units called volts: 1 volt = 1 joule/coulomb where a joule is a unit of energy and a coulomb is a unit of charge (1 coulomb = 6×10^{18} electrons).

The movement or flow of electric charge from one point in a system to another point is called *current*, abbreviated I. Current flows only if there is a potential difference between two points, that is, only if we have separation of charge (i.e., voltage). Current (I) is measured in amperes, 1 ampere = 1 coulomb/sec.

When charge moves in a medium, for example, in a solution or in a wire, the medium tends to hinder or retard the flow of charge. How much it hinders charge flow depends on the nature of the material. For example, copper wire (a conductor) does not hinder the movement of charge to any appreciable extent, whereas rubber (an insulator) greatly restricts charge movement. This restriction or hindrance to the movement of charge offered by a material is called *resistance*. The amount of current that flows depends on the resistance of the material through which it is flowing. The greater the resistance, the less the amount of current that will flow if voltage is held constant. Resistance is measured in *ohms*. Thus, the amount of current that flows between two points in a medium depends on the voltage separating the two points and the resistance of the medium through which it flows. Ohm's Law relates voltage (E), current (I), and resistance (R): E = IR or I = E/R. By holding one parameter constant and measuring another we can calculate the third.

One other element of electricity that we must consider before discussing the passive electrical properties of biological membranes is *capacitance*, the ability to store and separate charges. In electrical circuits, a capacitor is composed of two parallel conducting plates separated by an insulator. A capacitor can store electric charge on its plates but charge cannot pass through the barrier of insulation. The closer together the two plates are, and the larger the plates, the greater the capacity to store and separate charge, and the greater the capacitance. Capacitance is measured in units called *farads*. One farad is the capacity to hold 1 coulomb with a potential difference between the two plates of 1 volt. In electrical circuits and in biological membranes, capacitance slows the flow of electrical charges. It therefore introduces the element of time into changes in potential and the flow of current.

Biological membranes in general and neuronal membranes in particular have resistance and a capacitance; they limit and slow changes in potential and the flow of current. For example, if we apply a potential difference (i.e., a voltage) across a biological membrane (e.g., a

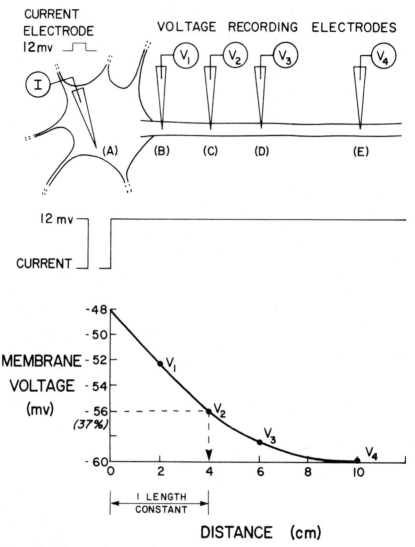

Figure 4. Neuron showing the decline over distance of an applied voltage and illustrating the length constant of the membrane.

nerve fiber) at point A, and measure the voltage at increasing distances away from point A, we would discover that the amount of voltage decreased as the distance from point A increased. An example of such an experiment is shown in Figure 4. How much the voltage declines is a function of the membrane. A measure of this decline over distance of an applied voltage is the *length, or space, constant* of the membrane, abbreviated λ (Lamda). The length constant is the distance over which an applied voltage declines to approximately one-third its original value. For example, in Figure 4 current is injected to change the membrane potential +12 mV at point A. At point B, 2 cm away, the recording electrode measures *not* 12 mV, but rather 8 mV. At point C, 4 cm away from point A, 4 mV are measured. In this case, because the initial voltage is 12 mV, a decline to one-third of this value would give a voltage of $1/3 \times 12 = 4$ mV. This voltage occurred at 4 cm away from point A. Therefore, the length constant for this region of membrane is 4 cm. Length constants vary from neuron to neuron and are thought to vary along given sections of a particular neuron. The length constant is a useful measure because it tells us how one neuron compares to another with respect to the spread of voltage. In addition, it tells us how one synaptic input to a neuron can be much more effective in evoking a response than an identical but more distant input. Length constants explain the integrative phenomenon of spatial summation (described later in this chapter) whereby simultaneous subthreshold excitatory inputs to a neuron which occur at different regions on the neuronal membrane can sum to threshold level and initiate an action potential.

Just as the length constant tells us how far along a membrane an applied voltage will spread, the time constant τ (Tau) is defined as the time it takes an applied voltage to increase to 63% (about two-thirds) of its final value (Fig. 5). In Figure 5, this is equal to 50 ms; the time it takes the membrane potential to reach 63% of its final value of 10 mV. Time constants are, in part, a measure of membrane capacitance, which are useful when considering the integrative mechanism of temporal summation. Here, subthreshold excitatory inputs that occur close together in time can sum to threshold, causing a response. The behavioral significance of the integrative mechanisms of spatial and temporal summation will be discussed later in this chapter. What is important to recognize here is that all nerve membranes both limit the spread of charge and slow down such electrotonic spread. Yet each neuronal membrane has its own characteristic way of doing this. The length constant and time constant are best understood when one thinks of them as quantitative descriptions of differences among neurons with respect to how they limit and slow the spread of electrical charges.

The Resting Membrane Potential

If a suitable microelectrode is inserted into a cell (nerve or otherwise), another electrode placed outside of the cell in the extracellular environment, and the two electrodes connected to a voltmeter, a potential difference on the order of millivolts (mV, 10^{-3} V) will be measured (Fig. 6). This potential difference between the inside and outside of a cell is called the *resting membrane potential* and is generally negative

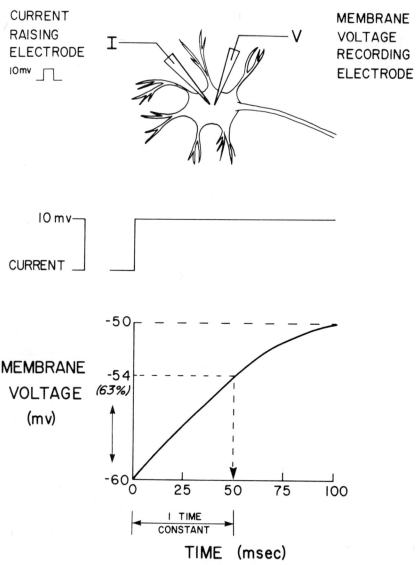

Figure 5.   Neuron showing the rise over time of an applied voltage and illustrating the time constant of the membrane.

inside with respect to the outside. Resting potentials are time-independent potentials, that is, they do not vary from minute to minute, or hour to hour, but are generally constant. All cells have a resting potential whose magnitude varies between −5 and −100 mV depending on the cell type. Most nerve cells have resting membrane potentials on the order of −70 to −100 mV inside negative.

Resting potentials originate because of differences in the ionic com-

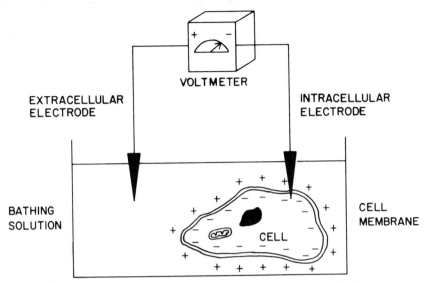

Figure 6.   The measurement of the resting membrane potential of a cell.

position between the fluid of the extracellular environment and that
of the intracellular environment, and because of the nature of the cell
membrane that separates these two environments. The origin of the
cell resting membrane potential is perhaps easiest to understand by
considering a simple case where two ionic solutions of similar but *not*
identical composition are separated by a barrier that is freely and
equally permeable to all ion species in the two solutions (Fig. 7). In
Figure 7, the solution on side 1 contains 0.1 M NaCl, a tenfold higher
concentration than the solution on side 2. Because the barrier is freely
permeable to all ionic species and because sodium and chloride are in
higher concentration on side 1, both Na+ and Cl− ions will move
from side 1 to side 2, down their respective concentration gradient.
However, because chloride in a water environment has a smaller
effective diameter than sodium, it will move from side 1 to side 2 at a
faster rate. Therefore, for a brief time, side 2 will have an excess of
negatively charged chloride ions (*panel* B). Solution 2 will therefore be
negative with respect to solution 1. We have established a potential
difference between side 1 and side 2. Eventually, the negativity of
side 2 will retard the movement of chloride, but accelerate the movement of sodium. With time, the rates of movement of the two ion
species will become equal and the concentration of sodium and chloride will be the same. At this point, no potential difference will exist.

   In Figure 8, the 0.01 M NaCl solution on side 2 has been replaced by
a 0.1 M KCl solution. Side 1 therefore resembles the extracellular
fluid—it is high in sodium whereas side 2 now resembles the intracel-

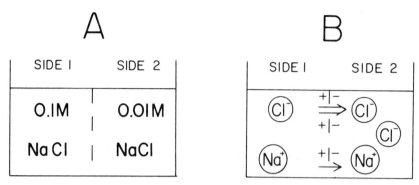

Figure 7. Ionic charge movements across a freely permeable membrane.

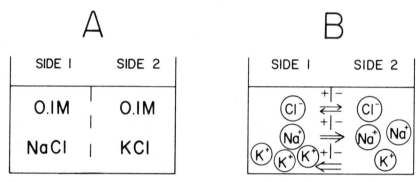

Figure 8. Charge movements across a *freely* permeable membrane with solutions resembling extracellular and intracellular fluids.

lular fluid, it is high in potassium. In this case, sodium ions will move down their concentration gradient from side 1 to side 2. Likewise, potassium ions will move down their concentration gradient from side 2 to side 1. Because chloride ions are in equal concentration on each side (i.e., no concentration gradient), there will be no *net* movement of chloride. Because potassium ions move faster than sodium ions, side 1 will develop a temporary excess of positively charged potassium ions and become positive (+) with respect to side 2. As in Figure 7, a potential difference will now exist between side 1 and side 2, with side 1 being positive with respect to side 2. Again, with time, an equilibrium condition will be reached and the difference in potential will disappear.

As a final example, we will change the nature of the barrier that separates side 1 from side 2 to one that allows the potassium ions to cross, but does *not* allow sodium ions to cross (i.e., it is permeable to potassium but impermeable to sodium). In this case, we will observe the following behavior (Fig. 9A). Potassium ions will move from side 2 to side 1, down their concentration gradient, but sodium ions are

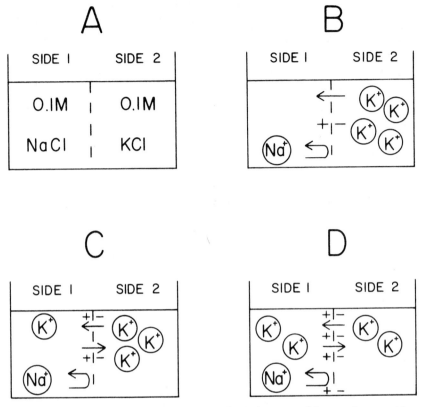

Figure 9. Charge movements across a *selectively* permeable membrane with solutions resembling extracellular and intracellular fluids.

unable to move because the membrane restricts them to their original side, side 1 (Fig. 9B). Therefore, side 1 gains positive potassium ions and a potential difference starts to develop. However, the positivity of side 1 will start to repel the movement of potassium, whereas the negativity of side 2 will attract potassium ions. Therefore, some potassium will move back from side 1 to side 2 (Fig. 9C). Eventually, the potential difference will be large enough to oppose any further *net* movement of potassium into side 1. At this point, the force of the electrical potential difference is equal and opposite to the force of the concentration gradient. And, at this point, the amount of potassium entering side 2 will be equal to the amount leaving side 1 (Fig. 9D).

In each of the above cases, the force responsible for the *net* movement or diffusion of the ions is the difference in concentration between side 1 and side 2. As this concentration force moves ions from one side to another, a potential difference or voltage develops. This potential difference then begins to influence the movement of the ions. Positively charged ions like potassium and sodium are attracted to areas of negativity and repelled by areas of positivity. This force of attraction between unlike charges and force of repulsion between like charges is the electrical force. Once it becomes equal to the force resulting from differences in concentration for an ion, net movement of the ion will cease (Fig. 9 D). At *equilibrium potential* (E_{ion}) for the ion in question, there is no *net* movement of the ion because the force of concentration gradients is exactly balanced by the potential difference created across the two sides of a barrier. The magnitude of the equilibrium potential for an ion depends primarily on the concentration gradient; the greater this gradient, the greater is the equilibrium potential. This potential for an ion can be determined if the concentrations of the ion on either side of a barrier or membrane are known. In nerve cells, the equilibrium for potassium is about -75 mV inside negative, whereas that for sodium is about $+50$ mV inside positive. Equilibrium potentials for various ionic species vary in both magnitude and direction depending on the concentration gradients.

It is now possible to explain the origin of the cell resting membrane potential. In a nerve cell at rest, the concentration of potassium ions inside is much greater than the concentration outside. Likewise, the concentration of sodium outside is much greater than that inside. Second, the nerve cell membrane at rest is some 50 to 75 times more permeable to potassium than to sodium. Therefore, potassium ions will diffuse out of the cell down their concentration gradients so that the inside of the nerve cell becomes negative with respect to the outside. Eventually, the net movement of potassium will stop when the potential difference across the nerve cell membrane is equal and opposite to the force produced by the concentration gradient. This occurs near the potassium equilibrium potential. For most nerve cells, the resting membrane potential that is measured by intracellular microelectrode is somewhat less negative than the potassium equilibrium potential, because the cell membrane is not completely impermeable to sodium ions. Thus, some sodium ions leak into the cell, adding positive ions to the cell interior and keeping the resting membrane potential somewhat less negative than the potassium equilibrium potential. And, because the cell resting potential is *not* exactly at the potassium equilibrium potential, there is a continual *net* movement of potassium ions out of the cell and a small leak of sodium ions into the cell.

The concentration gradients for sodium and potassium ions do not run down with time because of an active-transport mechanism located in the cell membrane of the nerve cell. This mechanism uses energy derived from cellular metabolism to pump potassium ions back into the cell and sodium ions out. In most nerve cells the pumping of these two ions occurs in a way that does not make a direct contribution to the separation of charge. This membrane pump is responsible for maintaining the concentration gradients across the cell membrane and is found in virtually all cells. It is called the sodium-potassium pump and owes its pumping ability to its adenosine triphosphatase (ATPase) activity. This enzymatic activity enables the pump to split ATP to adenosine diphosphate (ADP) thereby yielding energy from the broken high energy bond. The energy required to drive the $Na+/K+$ pump mechanism in each of the millions of individual nerve cells in the nervous system accounts for the major expenditure of energy by this system.

Action Potentials

In our discussion of the resting membrane potential, we saw that one of its main characteristics is its constancy. As long as the permeability of the cell membrane barrier does not change and as long as the concentration gradients are maintained, the resting membrane potential is steady. Changes in the membrane potential away from its resting value are used by cells to convey information about changes in the extracellular or intracellular environment. Nerves and other electrically excitable cells such as muscle cells have capitalized on this and use changes in resting membrane potential for transmitting, receiving, and integrating information. These changes in resting potential are of two types: *graded* and *all-or-none action* potentials. Graded potentials occur primarily at synapses (the point of contact between a nerve and its effector cell) and at the specialized endings of sensory receptors where the distances over which information is passed are short. Graded membrane potential changes will be discussed in the section concerning synaptic transmission.

Action potentials are used by the nervous system to convey information over relatively long distances. Action potentials are extremely fast changes in the resting membrane potential, on the order of 1 to 10 ms (1 ms $= 1 \times 10^{-3}$). During this time, the resting membrane potential goes from a value of some -70 mV through zero to $+30$ mV and then rapidly to -70 mV (Fig. 10). How cells are able to do this and the ionic basis of the action potential will be discussed in the following section. First however, it is important to list the characteristics of action potentials along with the features that clearly distinguish them from graded potentials.

By definition, action potentials are time dependent, *all-or-none*, fixed amplitude, propagated waves of electrical activity. Action potentials are time dependent because they occur as discrete events, each of which can be described as occupying a brief interval of real time. They are all-or-none because once a threshold level is reached (e.g., by application of the appropriate stimulus) an action potential is generated. If stimulus strength is increased beyond threshold, the

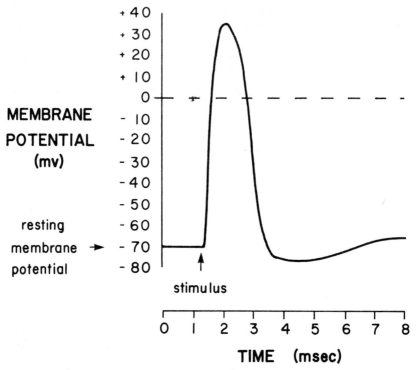

Figure 10. The changes in membrane potential associated with a single action potential.

size or amplitude of the action potential will remain the same. In other words, the size of the action potential is determined solely by the properties of the cell and is independent of the stimulus. Moreover, the amplitude of the action potential is constant. That is to say, the size of the action potential produced at the point of stimulation is identical to the size of the action potential that reaches some distant site in the nerve cell. Action potentials are also propagated along the cell membrane from one point to another. It is this property that allows the nervous system to use action potentials to convey information over long distances. For example, it is action potentials that convey stretch information from the tapped tendon of the knee to the spinal cord. And it is action potentials, initiated by the motor neuron and carried via its axon, that initiate the contraction of the quadriceps muscle.

Ionic Basis of the Action Potential

The underlying ionic mechanisms of the action potential were first detailed by English scientists, A.L. Hodgkin and A.F. Huxley, during the 1950s. For their work they received the Nobel Prize in 1963.

Action potentials can be explained using the concepts we have discussed for resting potentials. Remember that in nerve cells the resting membrane potential (−70 mV) is close to the equilibrium potential (−75 mV) for potassium and reflects the fact that (1) the cell membrane at rest is permeable to potassium but relatively impermeable to sodium; thus, there is a steady outward current of potassium and a small inward leak of sodium, and (2) sodium is high in concentration outside the cell. Also recall that the equilibrium potential for an ion is that potential which exactly opposes the force due to the concentration gradient. Once the membrane potential of the cell reaches the equilibrium potential, there will be no further *net* movement of the ion. However, until that level of membrane potential is reached, the force resulting from the concentration gradient will govern the movement of the ion.

During the action potential, these principles also apply; action potentials result from a transient change in the permeability of the cell membrane. During the rising phase of the action potential, the membrane becomes highly permeable to sodium (an increase of some 300 times) and sodium rushes into the cell. This is because its concentration gradient is directed inward and its equilibrium potential is near +50 mV (inside positive). During this time, there are more sodium ions entering the cell than potassium ions leaving; thus the cell depolarizes and the membrane potential goes from a resting value of −70 mV (inside negative) to approximately +30 mV (inside positive), approaching the sodium equilibrium potential. At this point, the permeability of the cell membrane again changes. The increased permeability to sodium that characterized the rising phase is rapidly shut off and the permeability to potassium is markedly increased above the resting level. These changes in membrane permeability drastically reduce the net inward movement of sodium ions and increase the net outward movement of potassium. During the falling phase of the action potential, there are more positive potassium ions leaving the cell interior than sodium ions entering. Therefore, the cell interior loses positively charged ions and thus becomes more negative. This continues until the resting potential level is reached. In fact, the membrane potential is restored to a value somewhat more negative than the initial resting potential. This after-hyperpolarization (or increase in negativity beyond resting level) is due to the fact that after the permeability to sodium has returned to resting level, the membrane permeability to potassium is still high. Eventually, the potassium permeability returns to its resting level and the resting membrane potential is restored. These changes all occur in less than 10 ms. The timing of these various events is shown in Figure 11. In considering the ionic movements during the action potential, it is important to understand that the fluxes of sodium and potassium across the cell membrane

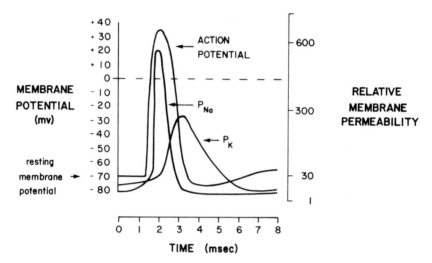

Figure 11.   Changes in permeability to sodium (P_{Na}) and potassium (P_K) during an action potential.

actually involve an extremely *small* number of ions. The actual number of ions that move is so small that there is virtually no change in
the concentration gradient during an action potential. With time however, and after a large number of action potentials, the concentration
gradients for sodium and potassium would change were it not for the
membrane pump. Thus, while the sodium-potassium pump plays no
direct role in the generation of the action potential, it does maintain
the concentration gradients constant over time.

The mechanisms responsible for changing membrane permeability
are not well understood. We know, however, that these mechanisms
are sensitive to the electrical potential difference across the cell membrane. The permeability of the cell membrane to sodium ions is
increased by depolarization, that is, by making the membrane potential less negative (i.e., closer to zero) than its resting value. Hyperpolarization (making it more negative than the resting value), on the
other hand, decreases the permeability to sodium. It is this effect of
membrane potential on membrane permeability to sodium ions that
accounts for the explosive, all-or-none nature of the action potential.
Appropriate stimulation results in a depolarization of the cell membrane. This increases the membrane's permeability to sodium. Therefore, more positive Na+ ions flow into the cell. This inward flow of
positive ions in turn produces a greater depolarization. Greater depolarization causes an even larger increase in the membrane's permeability to sodium (Fig. 12). Eventually, the sodium equilibrium
potential is approached and the process subsides. In addition, the
sodium permeability shuts down or is said to inactivate. With this

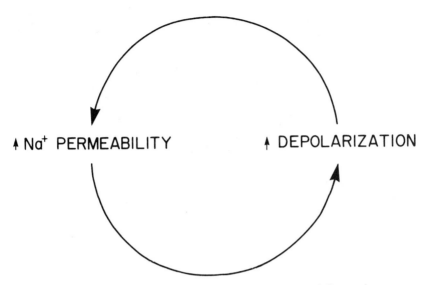

Figure 12.   Interactive effects of increased sodium permeability and depolarization during the rising phase of an action potential.

information we can explain many of the properties of action potentials.

THRESHOLD

Action potentials occur only if the resting membrane potential is suffi-ciently depolarized so that the influx of sodium exceeds the efflux of potassium ions. The membrane potential at which this occurs is called the *threshold potential* or the critical membrane potential. For most nerve cells, the threshold potential is some 5 to 15 mV less negative than the resting potential. Weak depolarizations that do not reach the threshold potential are called subthreshold (and the stimuli that pro-duce them, subthreshold stimuli). These do not produce an action potential. Strong depolarizations that go beyond the threshold poten-tial are called suprathreshold and elicit an action potential of exactly the same size as a threshold stimulation.

REFRACTORY PERIODS

If a second threshold stimulus is applied immediately following the generation of an action potential initiated by a threshold stimulus, the cell membrane may not always respond. Even though identical stim-uli are applied each time, the membrane is unresponsive or *refractory* to a second stimulus. If we increase the second stimulus to well above threshold levels (i.e., make it suprathreshold), we can produce an action potential. This period of reduced responsiveness immediately following the generation of an action potential is called the *relative refractory* period. During this time, the membrane's permeability to potassium is still above the resting level. Thus, a depolarization of greater than threshold value is required for sodium ions to enter the cell in sufficient number to counteract the increased potassium efflux. The application of a second stimulus *during* the action potential depolarization will not produce a second action potential no matter how great the stimulus strength. This period of total unresponsiveness is called the *absolute refractory period* and it limits the number of action potentials that can be produced by a given nerve cell in a given period of time (i.e., it limits the frequency with which a neuron can produce action potentials).

PROPAGATION

An important property of action potentials is their propagation from one point to another. It is important to understand, however, that one action potential does not itself travel along the nerve cell membrane; instead, each action potential excites or triggers a new action potential in the adjacent areas of membrane. Recall that current flows wherever there is voltage. Local currents flow between the region where the depolarization of the action potential is occurring and the adjacent membrane which is at the resting membrane potential. This current flow causes these adjacent areas of membrane to become depolarized to threshold level. Once this level of membrane potential is reached, the all-or-none action potential is elicited in the area of membrane adjacent to the region where the action potential just occurred.

Because the area of membrane that has just undergone an action potential is, for a brief moment, refractory, the only direction of action potential propagation is away from the site of stimulation. A schematic representation of this is shown in Figure 13. How far in front of the action potential the local currents spread depends on the length constant of the membrane, which in turn depends on the resistance to current flow offered by the cell membrane and the intracellular and extracellular fluids. Generally, the greater the length constant, the faster the action potential propagation (i.e., greater conduction velocity). Larger diameter fibers offer less resistance to current flow. Because this is so, larger fibers have larger length constants and faster conduction velocities than fibers of smaller diameter.

Myelination of nerve fibers also greatly influences conduction velocity. Myelin is a lipid-rich material surrounding the axons of most

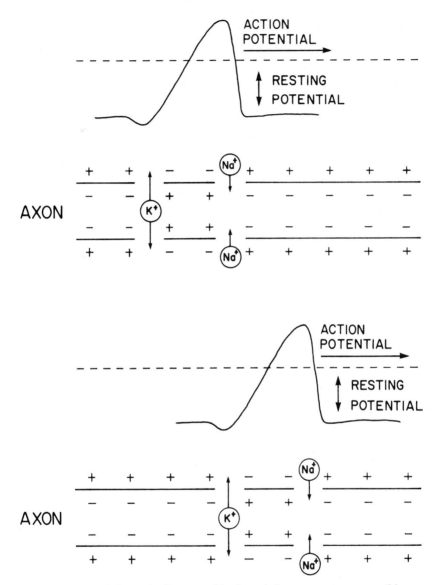

Figure 13. *Top:* Schematic diagram of ionic and charge events responsible for action potential propagation. *Bottom:* Shows state of same membrane a short time later to illustrate propagation of action potential.

neurons. Myelin electrically insulates the axon, making it much more difficult for current to flow between the intracellular and extracellular fluids. In effect, it increases the length constant and therefore there is less decrement in the voltage gradient along the membrane. Action potentials do not occur where there is myelin; they occur only where the myelin sheath is interrupted. These interruptions occur at regular intervals along the axon and are called nodes of Ranvier. Because action potentials occur only at the nodes, they appear to leap or jump from one node to the next. This type of action potential propagation is very fast (about 120 m/sec in a large myelinated fiber) and is called saltatory conduction.

Nerve cells convey information to three kinds of effector cells: nerve, muscle, and gland (e.g., chromaffin cells of the adrenal medulla). The point of communication between a nerve and its effector cell is called a synapse. The morphological and ultrastructural features of the various types of synapses have been discussed earlier. In this section, the mechanisms by which information is conveyed across the synapse are discussed.

Synaptic transmission was for many years believed to be purely electrical in nature because of the speed with which it occurs. A chemical basis for synaptic transmission is of two forms. "Electrical" transmission occurs in some central nervous system synapses and in many synapses in invertebrates, and second, there is "chemical" transmission—by far the most common form of synaptic transmission in mammals. For this reason, this discussion is restricted to chemical synaptic transmission. An earlier section on neuronal anatomy described the unique ultrastructure that is a synapse. There is a nerve ending or nerve terminal, as it is appropriately called, which is the specialized ending of an axon. Within the membrane surrounding the nerve terminal are many of the usual intracellular organelles including mitochondria, Golgi apparatus, microfilaments, and microtubules. In addition, there is a large population of synaptic vesicles, spherical structures containing an inner core surrounded by a distinct membrane. The nerve terminal is separated from the effector cell (which is called the postsynaptic cell) by a space or gap called the synaptic cleft. This space is generally filled with a fine amorphous material and is on the order of 10 nm wide. The postsynaptic cell immediately adjacent to the nerve terminal also has specializations in structure, the details of which depend upon its nature. These ultrastructural features are intimately related to the function of the synapse.

In chemical transmission, a chemical transmitter substance is stored in the vesicles of the nerve terminal. On command, it is released into the synaptic cleft and diffuses across the cleft to react with specialized sites on the postsynaptic cell. As a result of this interaction between the chemical transmitter and the specialized regions on the membrane a permeability change is produced. This permeability change in turn causes a redistribution of ions (i.e., current flow) producing a change in the resting membrane potential.

The paradigm for the study of chemical transmission is the frog neuromuscular junction. Primarily as a result of the work of Katz (1969) and his collaborators, we now understand much about the molecular events associated with transmission at this synapse in the peripheral nervous system.

In the following section, the events associated with chemical transmission are presented using the frog neuromuscular junction as an example. Although other synapses have been studied, none has been studied in such great detail. What we have learned from the frog neuromuscular junction seems to be applicable to chemical synapses in general.

The Steps in Chemical Transmission

1. Chemical transmission is initiated by the depolarization associated with the arrival of an action potential at the nerve terminal.

2. As a result of this change in membrane potential, the permeability of the nerve terminal membrane to calcium ions (Ca+) greatly increases. This permeability at rest is very low.

3. Because of the large, inwardly directed concentration gradient for calcium, which is reflected in its equilibrium potential (> 100 mV, inside positive), the driving force on calcium is large and thus, when the permeability of the membrane increases, calcium moves rapidly inward and a calcium current develops.

4. As a result of the inward movement of calcium, the concentration of free intracellular calcium increases and the vesicle contents of neurotransmitter, acetylcholine (ACh), in the case of the neuromuscular junction, are extruded to the extracellular space of the synaptic cleft. A single action potential is thought to cause some 200 or more synaptic vesicles to simultaneously release their content of transmitter substance into the synaptic cleft.

5. Once in the synaptic cleft, ACh has three possible fates: First, it may simply diffuse out of the cleft; second, it may be hydrolyzed rapidly to acetate + choline by the enzyme acetylcholinesterase (ACh-E) which is present in high concentration in the synaptic cleft. Or third, it can bind to a specialized receptor (ACh-R). In fact, all three events occur.

6. As a result of the binding of ACh to its receptor, it is believed that a change in conformation of the receptor occurs so that the permeability of the postsynaptic membrane to sodium and potassium increases.

7. This increase in permeability allows sodium to move inward, down its electrical and concentration gradients, and at the same time allows potassium to move out of the cell along its concentration and electrical gradient. These positive ions therefore move in opposite directions at the same time. Inasmuch as the sodium current is somewhat larger, the *net* current is inward. This results in a depolarization that lasts as long as the permeability of the postsynaptic membrane is increased. At the neuromuscular junction the depolarization that results from the release of ACh and its action at the postsynaptic membrane is called the *end-plate potential* (EPP). At other synapses it is a *postsynaptic potential* (PSP).

8. At the neuromuscular junction, the EPP is normally of sufficient size to cause a depolarization of the adjacent muscle fiber membrane to beyond the threshold potential, resulting in a muscle action potential and muscle contraction.

9. The ACh is bound to its receptor only for a brief period. It quickly dissociates from the receptor and is hydrolyzed by the esterase enzyme, ACh-E. Once ACh is removed from the receptor, the permeability to sodium and potassium decreases quickly back to resting levels. Thus, unlike the action potential, the EPP decays passively from its most depolarized state back to the resting potential as a result of the dissociation of ACh from its receptor.

We have seen what happens at the presynaptic nerve terminal when the nerve is stimulated and an action potential invades the nerve terminal. However, at the neuromuscular junction, and presumably at all other chemical synapses, there is spontaneous release of transmitter that results in a very small (mean amplitude of 0.5 mV) depolarization of the postsynaptic membrane. These small depolarizations resemble the much larger EPP and are therefore called *miniature end-plate potentials* or MEPPs. Each MEPP is thought to be the result of the random, spontaneous leakage of the contents of a single presynaptic vesicle and is called a *quantum unit* of release because it is the smallest quantity of transmitter that can be released. The mechanism by which the synaptic vesicle extrudes its contents of transmitter to the extracellular environment is called exocytosis. This mechanism is now thought to be the common cellular mechanism of secretion where a prepackaged product (that is stored within a vesicle) is destined for export. Studies by Douglas (1968), Foreman and Mongar (1975), and others have shown that calcium ions are a necessary prerequisite for exocytosis, the process by which intracellular material is carried within vesicles to the cell surface where it fuses with the plasma membrane and then breaks down to release its contents into the extracellular region. Douglas has suggested that the rise in the level of free intracellular calcium initiates exocytosis. This mechanism of secretion involves the movement of the vesicle to the

PRESYNAPTIC NERVE TERMINAL

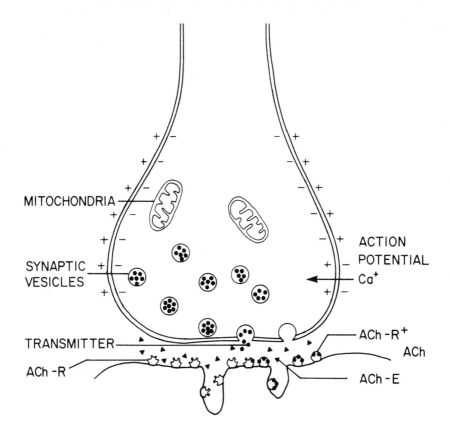

Figure 14.   Representation of exocytotic release of neurotransmitter (ACh), depolarization by esterase (ACh-E) and receptor (ACh-R) binding postsynaptically (ACh-R + ACh).

cell membrane, the fusion of the cell membrane with the vesicle membrane, and the eventual rupture of this fused membrane. This results in the externalization of the vesicle contents. At the neuromuscular junction, recent evidence suggests that exocytosis occurs at specific sites along the inside of the nerve terminal membrane facing the synaptic cleft. These regions are called active zones. Interestingly, the active zones are located across the synaptic cleft from the tips of folds in the postsynaptic membrane (the junction folds); regions that have the highest density of ACh receptor. The steps involved in chemical transmission are summarized in Figure 14.

As shown in Figure 14, the presynaptic neurons influence postsynaptic cells (neurons, muscle cells, or gland cells) by means of chemical transmitters. In the preceding discussion, ACh and the neuromuscular junction were used as an example to explain the process of chemical transmission. At the neuromuscular junction, ACh is an example of an excitatory transmitter causing excitation of skeletal muscle fibers. In the central nervous system, there are many other known or suspected excitatory neurotransmitters. These include norepinephrine and epinephrine, dopamine, serotonin (5-hydroxtriptamine), histamine, and many neuropeptides (Cooper et al. 1978). Of course, these transmitters may not be excitatory under *all* circumstances because the receptor complex has a profound effect on the nature of the transmitter's response. Although the general mechanisms involved in chemical transmission at CNS synapses are believed to be the same as those occurring at the neuromuscular junction, there are exceptions. For example, central synapses of the mammalian nervous system are considerably more complicated than the neuromuscular junction because several (from a few to a thousand) presynaptic nerve terminals end on a single neuron. An example of this is the spinal motor neuron of the cat, which has been studied in some detail by Eccles (1964), where many hundreds of presynaptic fibers end on a single motor neuron. Stimulation of excitatory presynaptic nerve terminals produces a graded potential in the motor neuron called the *excitatory postsynaptic potential* (EPSP). It is analogous to the EPP of the neuromuscular junction. The major differences are: (1) The EPSP is much smaller in amplitude and therefore it generally requires the summation of several EPSPs to excite the motor neuron. By stimulating a larger number of presynaptic fibers, the amplitude of the EPSP increases. (2) The permeability change in the postsynaptic membrane of the motor neuron that is responsible for the EPSP is to all small ions—predominantly $Na+$, $K+$, and $Cl-$, and not just $Na+$ and $K+$ as occurs at the neuromuscular junction.

In addition to excitatory chemical transmission, there is also *inhibitory* chemical transmission. In mammalian nervous systems, inhibitory neurotransmitters generally occur at central nervous system synapses. Again, the spinal motor neuron can also serve as an example of an inhibitory synapse. Some presynaptic fibers exert an inhibitory influence on the motor neuron and thus tend to reduce its firing rate. As with central excitatory neurotransmission, the same principles of chemical transmission apply: the neurotransmitter is released from the presynaptic nerve terminal, binds to some receptor molecule on the postsynaptic membrane, and, as a result of this binding, the permeability of the postsynaptic membrane is altered. For inhibitory neurotransmitters, the permeability change generally results in a hyperpolarization, thereby moving the membrane potential further away from the threshold potential. The best known and most studied inhibitory transmitter substance is gamma amino butyric acid or GABA (Kuffler and Edwards 1958). This is an inhibitory transmitter at crustacean neuromuscular junctions and is strongly suspected of being an inhibitory transmitter in the mammalian central nervous system. When GABA binds to its postsynaptic membrane receptor, it causes an increase in the membrane's permeability to chloride ions. The resulting potential change is called an *inhibitory postsynaptic potential* (IPSP). Like the EPSP, it is a local, graded potential whose decay depends upon the dissociation of transmitter from receptor and whose amplitude depends on the number of inhibitory presynaptic nerve terminals firing.

Another form of inhibition is *presynaptic inhibition*. In this case an inhibitory synapse is located on an excitatory presynaptic nerve terminal. The effect of presynaptic inhibition is to reduce the amount of excitatory transmitter substance that is released. To do this, it is necessary for the presynaptic inhibitory transmitter to be released before stimulation of the excitatory nerve terminal. Presynaptic inhibition selectively eliminates or reduces specific inputs to a neuron without affecting other inputs.

Neural Integration and Behavior

It should be apparent from the preceding discussion of EPSPs and IPSPs that information relayed across a synapse from one neuron to another is not propagated by the postsynaptic neuron in a form identical to that transmitted along the presynaptic neuron's axon. It is characteristic of neurons that they not only *receive* information, but also modify and transmit such information to other neurons and effector organs. Sensory receptors illustrate this principle. When stimuli in the form of light, mechanical displacement, or chemical agents impinge upon the terminal receptor elements of sensory (afferent) neurons they are *transduced* or *encoded* as patterns of neural activity. In other words, the various stimuli reaching the sensory receptors are transformed into patterns of action potentials, the electrical language of the nervous system. As noted earlier, the configuration and size of each action potential is determined solely by the properties of the cell and is independent of the stimulus. It is the temporal and spatial patterning of action potentials that convey information about the external and internal environment.

The transformation of stimuli into action potentials is accomplished by a stimulus-induced change in the membrane potential of the sensory receptor. This potential change is called a *generator potential*. Generator potentials initiate action potentials by depolarizing the membrane adjacent to the sensory receptor to its threshold level. Generator potentials are local, graded potentials that are spread passively for very short distances along the receptor terminal to a region where the nerve fiber membrane has a low threshold for generating action potentials. This point is often at the first node of Ranvier. Here, action potentials arise and do so with a frequency proportional to the stimulus intensity. Weak stimuli that produce small subthreshold generator potentials may not give rise to any action potentials. Brief, stronger stimuli give rise to large generator potentials and may initiate one or more action potentials. Stronger stimuli that are maintained for some time may generate long trains of action potentials. Because the frequency of action potential discharge conveys information concerning stimulus intensity or strength, such information is said to be *frequency coded*. In general, an increase in the frequency of firing of an afferent neuron is usually a signal that the intensity of stimulation has increased. The pattern of specific interneuronal synapses and the somatotopic specificity with which information from peripheral receptors project to higher centers such as the thalamus and cortex permit the accurate localization of stimuli. Such anatomic precision in ascending pathways leads us to describe stimulus localization as being *place coded*. That is to say, the thalamic and cortical neurons which respond to a given stimulus receive information from only a very highly localized portion of the body. In addition to stimulus location being place coded, it appears that the stimulus modality or type of stimulus is also place coded. Afferent information from a particular region of the body projects both to a specific cortical region corresponding to that body region and within this given cortical area to a region corresponding to one particular kind of sensory information.

Although important stimulus information is transduced at sensory receptors and coded into action potentials that are a neuronal "language," such information is always a modification of the original stimulus energy and never an exact copy. The output signals of sensory neurons that are propagated and coded by both frequency and place are never identical to the input signals that reach the receptor. This process in its most general form is termed "integration." With respect to the nervous system, integration is defined as those mechanisms or processes whereby the output signals of single cells or assemblies of cells is determined as a function of their input signals (Bullock 1977). Processes that modify *incoming* information to the nervous system are termed "sensory integration." Sensory integration usually transforms information about the external and internal environments into a selective and simplified, yet meaningful, representation of events. Through this process, information most useful to the individual is preserved. Information that is of little value is either not encoded at all or is minimally preserved.

Pause and consider your own brain. It resides suspended in cerebrospinal fluid, floating within the dark vault that is your cranium. Its only awareness of the outside world is via those afferent neurons capable of transducing environmental energies into nervous excitation. Your brain has never truly *seen* the light of day, nor has it *smelled* a rose, nor *touched* the grass. All that your brain believes that it knows about your world is to some extent a marvelous illusion. Your brain creates a model or abstraction of reality that is neither a lie nor the truth. It is not a lie because each nervous system extracts certain important information out of the flux of environmental energy and uses this information to help you survive, to thrive, and importantly to reproduce and continue your species. But the brain can by no means know of all reality surrounding our bodies. It sees neither x-rays nor infrared. It cannot feel the molecules of the air. Your brain is only concerned with certain *salient features* of the world that help you to guide your behavior toward adaptive, i.e., survival oriented and reproductive success.

Your brain makes up only about 2% of your total body weight, yet it demands almost 15% of your total cardiac output and close to 20% of the oxygen you use. Clearly, your brain uses a disproportionate amount of the energy resources of your body. The vast majority of the energy used by the brain is needed to maintain the resting membrane potentials of the billions of neurons.

Evolution has dictated that the brain not contain too many neurons, nor extract and process too much information. In fact, it is the role of the brain to *select, edit,* and *sample* events in the physical world and present an accurate but incomplete view of reality to your mind. Further increases in brain size would dictate that increasingly larger amounts of time be spent at searching for food and eating just to supply the brain with nutrients. There would also be considerable increases in the demands placed on heart and lungs to provide oxygen for the brain.

Hard as it may be to accept, the brain has made the best decision by *not* being able to provide a total picture of reality. If one can accept that the brain lives in a dark box and only receives partial information about the environments in which the body resides, one can press forward and ask, "What are the mechanisms and processes that the nervous system uses to make reality meaningful to the brain?"

A simple genetically determined integrative mechanism for selectivity or decisionmaking at receptors is called *adaptation* (Fig. 15). Most receptors show decreased generator potentials (and hence a decreased frequency of action potentials) in response to continuous stimulation at a constant level. When this occurs, the receptor is said to *adapt*. Receptors such as the muscle spindle, pain receptors, temperature receptors, and certain joint position receptors are said to be *tonic receptors* (slowly adapting). In these receptors, a given frequency

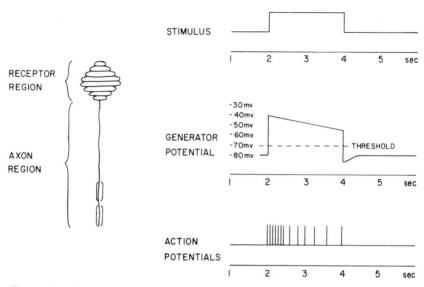

Figure 15.   Receptor adaptation showing how a constant stimulus gives rise to a generator potential that decays over time with resultant decrease in action potential frequency.

of action potentials will continue to be discharged at the receptor during periods of continuous stimulation from minutes to hours! Selective advantage to such prolongation of sensory activity is obvious. In the case of muscle spindles and joint receptors, slow adaptation allows for a *constant* monitoring of limb position and muscle tension even during constantly maintained loads, such as occur during activity requiring cocontraction or stabilization of a limb. If this were not the case, we would lose our awareness of the positions of body segments during activity where no motion occurs. For pain and temperature receptors, each of which signals impending or actual tissue damage, slow adaptation ensures that information concerning a noxious stimulus will be transmitted into the nervous system as long as it is present. This clearly impels us to take action to minimize or at least attend to such damage. If nociceptors adapted rapidly, we would soon become unaware of such destruction and perhaps fail to take appropriate action.

Other receptors such as those sensitive to the mechanical energy of touch and pressure are said to be *phasic receptors* (rapidly adapting). In less than a second, the generator potential decays and the receptor ceases firing action potentials when presented with a constant stimulus. This permits a high degree of sensitivity to changing stimuli but leads to a lack of awareness of constant inputs. For example, as you read this line, such rapid adaptation allows you to focus your attention on this text rather than on the sensations produced on your body surface by the chair in which you are sitting or the clothing you are wearing. In short, phasic receptors allow us to ignore constant stimuli that demand no immediate response and to attend quickly to changes in stimulus levels that do require immediate response. In contrast, tonic receptors permit you to attend to stimuli that are constant, yet would be maladaptive (a threat to survival) to ignore. Receptor adaptation depends on mechanical and biochemical properties of receptors. These remain quite stable over time. Even though sensory receptors do *integrate* information in the strict sense of the term, it is the more complex integrative processes that are commonly thought of as integrative events by most therapists. Consideration of sensory-motor integration is therefore a logical point of expansion of this discussion.

Sensory integrative events have received considerable attention from therapists recently. Those working with learning-disabled children are undoubtedly aware of the work of Ayres (1972, 1974, 1976, 1980) and her followers. However, even the the simplest reflex arc requires not only information processing by *afferent* neurons, but also by *efferent* neurons that allow for the expression of responses via muscular contractions and/or glandular secretions. At this point, it will be helpful to return to the earlier example of the alpha motor neuron (Figure 2). Simple examples are needed to describe integrative events that are typically present in this neuron as well as at other postsynaptic sites.

Temporal summation and spatial summation are two important integrative mechanisms (Figs. 16 and 17). When EPSPs (or IPSPs) are produced, they quickly attenuate. If a second EPSP is produced *at the same synapse* before the previous one has decayed, they *sum* together and produce a greater net membrane depolarization at that point than either would produce alone. Likewise, IPSPs sum to produce a greater net hyperpolarization. This is *temporal summation.* Just how closely these must occur in time to "overlap" and sum to a greater depolarization is described by the *time constant of the membrane* (τ) discussed earlier. In terms of the effect that such a mechanism has on the outputs of a postsynaptic neuron (remember integrative mechanisms determine outputs of neurons as functions of inputs), it can be seen that the higher the *frequency* of excitatory input at a single synapse, the greater the depolarization produced postsynaptically. The greater this depolarization, the greater the probability of the postsynaptic neuron firing an action potential (i.e., "responding").

Figure 16 shows in the top tracing that two identical subthreshold stimuli applied at the same point of afferent input on the membrane, but spaced 6 ms apart, produce identical EPSPs at that point. Remember that the time constant describes how the spread of charge is slowed via membrane capacitance (charge storage). The applied

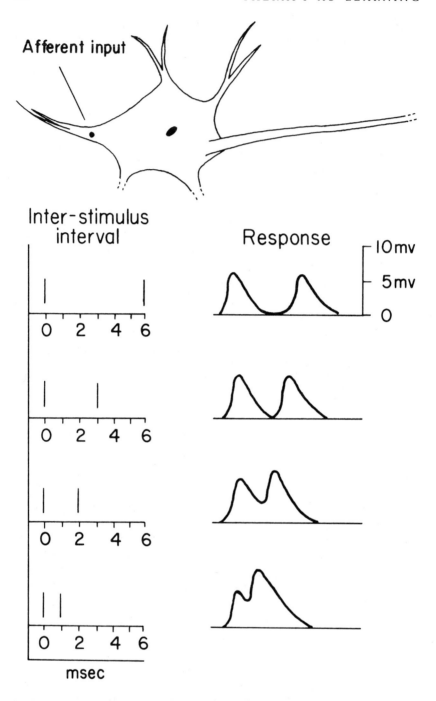

Temporal   Summation

Figure 16.   Diagram showing temporal summation.

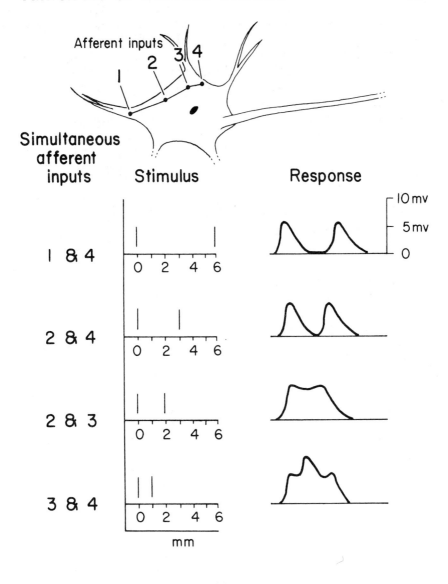

Spatial   Summation

Figure 17.   Diagram showing spatial summation.

charge stays briefly (in relation to neuronal time in which milliseconds represent entire events) and decays slowly. The second tracing shows that stimuli spaced 3 ms apart at the same point also produce identical amplitude EPSPs. However, the third tracing shows that if identical stimuli are given 2 ms apart at the same point, the amplitude of the second response EPSP is greater than the first. This is temporal summation, and the tracing at the bottom shows that even greater temporal summation takes place when identical stimuli occur only 1 ms apart at the same point. What has happened in these lower two tracings is that the capacitive properties of the membrane have "held" the charge briefly at the point of stimulation and maintained part of the stimulus-induced depolarization so that the second stimulus-induced depolarization does not depolarize the membrane from the resting condition. The likelihood of the membrane potential exceeding threshold and generating an action potential is thus enhanced by the closer temporal spacing of successive stimuli (i.e., increasing frequency of stimulation).

When EPSPs are produced at the same point in time, but at different points on the postsynaptic membrane, they too sum together and result in a larger net depolarization than would be produced by either alone. Inhibitory postsynaptic potential can also interact to produce greater net hyperpolarizations. These are examples of *spatial summation*. Just how closely together on the postsynaptic membrane these must occur to interact is described by the *length constant of the membrane* (λ).

Figure 17 shows in the top tracing that two identical subthreshold stimuli applied at the same point in time but spaced 7 mm apart produce identical EPSPs that fail to interact. The second and third tracings show that as simultaneous stimuli are placed closer together they eventually interact but fail to exceed the peak amplitude of EPSP depolarization induced by either alone. In the bottom tracing, however, when simultaneous stimuli spaced only 1 mm apart are observed, their EPSPs interact and sum to a greater net depolarization than either alone could produce. Remember that the length constant (λ) describes the gradual decay of charge across the membrane as a function of resistive properties. At 3 mm apart, each stimulus-induced depolarization decays to a net effect of zero halfway between the two points of application. At 2 mm or less apart, less charge loss occurs due to membrane resistance. Interactions of stimuli are therefore substantial. Once again, as is true with temporal summation, the likelihood of separate stimulus events interacting to produce a net depolarization to threshold and thus an action potential is enhanced by this mechanism.

Inasmuch as the typical motor neuron may receive input from up to 10,000 synapses, both the rate of presynaptic discharge and the location of synapses contribute to determine whether or not there will be action potentials discharged by the motor neuron. Because the axon hillock, a clearly recognizable elevation where the axon arises from the cell body of the neuron, typically has a relatively low threshold compared to the soma of the alpha motor neuron, inputs near this region have a greater influence (via temporal and spatial summation)

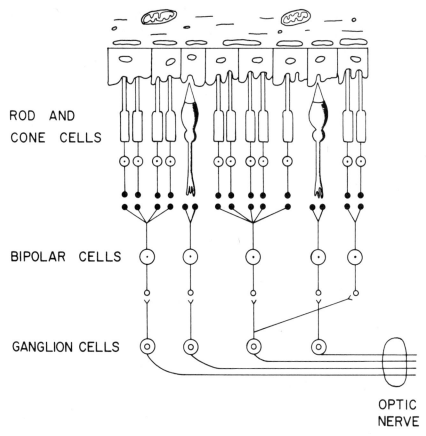

ROD AND CONE CELLS

BIPOLAR CELLS

GANGLION CELLS

OPTIC NERVE

Figure 18. Simplified diagram of neural convergence in the visual system.

over the response of the neuron than more remote inputs such as those on dendrites. This helps explain why proximal inputs to motor neurons such as the Renshaw cells (responsible for the recurrent inhibition of alpha motor neurons) are ideally located to produce maximal effects on the motor neuron.

Integration occurs not only within each neuron, but also between and among neurons. Although patterns of neuronal connectivity are often complex, several simple examples will serve to illustrate some integrative aspects of neuronal assemblies. *Neuronal convergence* serves to "focus" input from several to several thousand neuronal synapses on a single postsynaptic neuron. Most of these inputs are via synapses on the dendrites and soma of the neuron receiving such inputs. The visual system (Fig. 18) illustrates how a number of rods may send convergent input to a single retinal bipolar cell. Similarly, a number of bipolar cells all converge on a single retinal ganglion cell. Such a typical ganglion cell receives input from an average of 106 rod cells. There are about 120 million rods and 7 million cones in each retina. The optic nerve, comprised of ganglion cell axons, has but a million fibers. What does this convergence mean? Clearly, not all information that reaches the retina is preserved and conveyed in full detail. Ganglion cells, which receive inputs from rod cells (via bipolar cells), relay an integrated transformation of full visual detail into a somewhat simpler picture as represented in the optic nerve. At the fovea, where rod cells are absent, no convergence of cone cells is noted. Thus, all information received in this small zone is transmitted in full detail. Each foveal cone cell projects to a single bipolar cell, which in turn projects to a single ganglion cell. Because of this lack of convergence, the fovea is the region of greatest visual acuity.

The functional significance of neuronal convergence is twofold. First, it permits the "averaging" or "sampling" of a number of input sources to determine a simplified output. In this sense, convergence weeds out extraneous information. Second, convergence may permit a neuron or group of neurons to act as a decision-making or control unit. By comparing inputs from convergent presynaptic sources neurons may function as error-detectors or comparitors that measure discrepancies between expected feedback information and actual feedback. Such neurons may also issue output signals to minimize such input discrepancies. This occurs in the cerebellum and may allow for the comparison of intended movement results with actual feedback from ongoing movement and permit ongoing control of function as a result of a cerebellar decision as to whether results match intention.

Neuronal divergence (Fig. 19) is the reverse of convergence. Afferent or other neurons divide into numerous branches within the nervous system. Each branch may contribute excitatory or inhibitory inputs to more than 20,000 other neurons. Divergence, such as occurs in the dorsal column medial lemniscal system leads to a "spreading" of excitation. Tactile and proprioceptive information can thus be simultaneously transmitted to many regions of the nervous system including both conscious (cortex) and unconscious centers (cerebellum).

Divergence creates the possibility of different responses by various central nervous system (CNS) structures to a common source of input. Its functional significance is to allow for distributed (both in space and time) processing of information. Thus, each region of the CNS does not need its own receptors for each modality, but may still use the information from a given receptor in a way that differs from how another CNS region would use the same data.

One example of divergence which directly affects overt behavior is called *afterdischarge*. This integrative phenomenon is especially obvious in fast pain pathways (Fig. 20). A simple three-neuron reflex initiated by painful stimulation results in flexor muscles of a limb contracting and drawing the limb away from a noxious stimulus. This

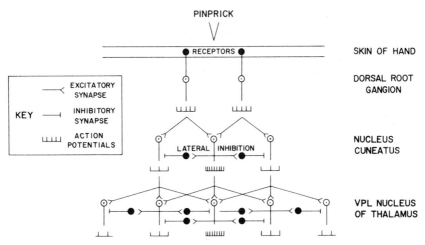

Figure 19.   Neuronal divergence as it occurs in the dorsal column/medial lemniscal pathway.

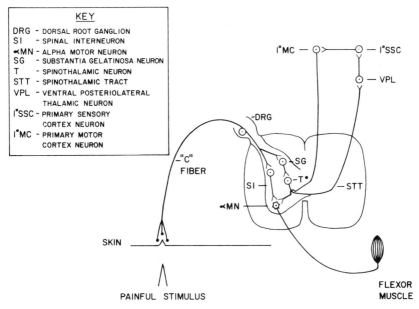

Figure 20.   Neuronal divergence in fast pain pathways using the phenomena of 'after discharge' as an example.

flexor withdrawal may last many milliseconds beyond termination of the painful stimulus. How does this happen? At the same time a direct three-neuron reflex initiates flexion, there is a divergence of pain information along multisynaptic pathways extending to the thalamus and cortex. Information is also projected via returning efferent signals to flexor muscles of the limb. The time required for the initiation of reflex withdrawal is the time needed to conduct the information along the three neurons and across the two synapses and the neuromuscular junction. Yet the divergence of such information over multisynaptic transcortical pathways ensures that the flexor alpha motor neurons will also receive cortical excitation at a time after the initial reflexive withdrawal. Because the flexor alpha motor neuron temporally summates inputs, it is likely that those inputs create a maintained withdrawal of the limb.

The integrative mechanisms cited here are but a few of the many currently described by neuroscientists. Although most or all of these may be relevant to an understanding of the neural basis of learning in full detail, it is beyond the scope of this work to fully describe these. These examples are provided because it is important to point out that the nervous system is not a passive relayer of information. It is first and foremost an information *processing* system. Inputs, be they information concerning bodily state or environmental changes, are modified and/or interpreted. Outputs (behaviors) are the product of neural events that take into account both present experience as well as the current state of the individual. Learning requires many such integrative events, yet not all such events lead to learning. Armed with the principles described in this chapter, the reader should now be prepared to examine the neurobiological bases of learning.

CHAPTER TWO

Learning Paradigms
and Neural Mechanisms

One difficulty that has faced therapists who have attempted to apply learning theories to clinical intervention is the lack of a systematic conceptual model or frame of reference that would permit a simplified yet accurate description of different kinds of learning. What has been missing is a descriptive typology of learning, the goal of which is to classify various types of learning with respect to dimensions that are clinically significant. The first criterion for a classification scheme was that it identify a means to relate clinical patterns of sensory stimulation with those patterns of action potentials known to induce changes in behavior. The second criterion was that this typology be able to rank these stimulation paradigms according to the longevity of the learned behavioral changes they evoke.

Kandel (1976:495) has said that "A learning paradigm describes how a stimulus must be patterned over time or combined with other stimuli to elicit specific modes of behavior." Six such paradigms of learning, which have relevance to therapy, are presented along with a review of current research findings concerning the neural mechanisms responsible for each type of learning.

We know that our experiences modify our abilities to respond and act and that only certain *patterns* of neural activity lead to changes in behavior. What neurobiologists and psychologists have come to appreciate is that, throughout development, stimuli that produce certain specific patterns of neural activity not only lead to behavioral change, but do so by modification of the *functional* strength of existing synaptic connections. Although anatomic plasticity of the nervous system plays a role in early maturation of neural pathways and in recovery from lesions, it appears that learning is primarily a process mediated by physiologic events, rather than by structural or anatomic changes. Six learning paradigms are presented in order of the longevity of their effects. Post-tetanic potentiation (PTP) and post-tetanic depression (PTD) are known to last from several minutes to several

41

hours and are therefore considered to be short-term learning phenomena. Habituation and sensitization effect behavioral changes, which last from hours to weeks. These are considered intermediate-term learning paradigms. Finally, classical and instrumental conditioning may be effective from weeks to years—in some cases, even for the lifetime of the individual. These, of course, are regarded as long-term learning.

In this section, each of six learning paradigms will be defined, followed by a behavioral description of this type of learning along with commentary on its adaptive significance. A description of the neural activity believed responsible for this phenomenon will also be presented. Next, four cellular mechanisms which are apparently responsible for physiologic modifications associated with learning will be discussed. Finally, the relevance of this six-paradigm typology of learning for therapists will be considered.

Two principles of neural systems are stressed. First, the nervous system does not transmit an exact duplicate of the sensory information which it receives. Sensory receptors *transform* environmental energy patterns into patterns of afferent nerve action potentials. Using vibration as an example, the actual mechanical displacement of the skin is a series of sinusoidal oscillations, whereas the action potentials arising from Pacinian corpuscles (vibration detectors) is a series of on and off bursts of action potentials. *The pattern and effects of afferent action potentials determine whether learning is going to occur*, not the pattern of environmental energy. In most cases the environmental pattern of stimulus energy and neural pattern of action potentials differ markedly.

Second, each individual neuron acts as an integrator of information. Whether a given neuron (afferent or efferent) fires is the result of interactions of all inputs as governed by the properties of the nerve cell membrane, and especially the length constant (λ), the time constant (τ), and the spatial distribution of inputs to that neuron. In clinical language these two principles imply:

1. Knowledge of environmental or clinically observable patterns of stimulation does not mean that resulting patterns of action potentials will be the same or even closely related. It is erroneous, therefore, to infer that action potential patterns resemble clinical stimulation patterns. Consider the rule stated by Farber (1982), that for facilitation to occur, "the rate of stimulation is generally fast, uneven and intermittent." Although often valid, the number of exceptions that represent inhibition rather than facilitation are unknown. More important is that such a rule does not account for underlying mechanisms and does not recognize that the neural patterning of action potentials in response to a stimulus determines whether or not learning will occur.

2. The effects of any specific pattern of stimulation depend on endogenous or "background" activity, all other inputs at the time, and the specific anatomic pathways involved.

SIX PARADIGMS OF LEARNING

If the various types of learning that are important for therapy are arranged in order of the expected longevity of behavioral changes they give rise to, the following sequence emerges:

Post-tetanic Potentiation (PTP)—minutes to hours
Post-tetanic Depression (PTD)—minutes to hours
Habituation—hours to weeks
Sensitization (Dishabituation)—hours to weeks
Classical Conditioning—up to years
Operant Conditioning—up to years

Each of these will now be described.

Post-tetanic potentiation (PTP) consists of repetitive high frequency stimulation of a neural pathway, resulting in an increase in the number of postsynaptic and/or muscle cells responding to a stimulus compared with responses to that stimulus seen before tetanization. With brief tetanization (10-15 sec), facilitation may last up to 3-4 min. With longer periods of tetanization (10-20 min), facilitation may last for several hours (Kandel 1976). Post-tetanic potentiation occurs not only at CNS synapses but also at the neuromuscular junction (Liley 1956).

Larrabee and Bronk (1947) reported that a 10-sec stimulation of a presynaptic fiber at a rate of 15 action potentials per second led to an increase in postsynaptic response magnitude which persisted approximately 3 min beyond the period of tetanic stimulation. Lloyd (1949) reported the occurrence of post-tetanic facilitation in the spinal cord of the cat as it affected the monosynaptic reflex responses of the gastrocnemius muscle.

An interesting and important feature of PTP is that the increase in response of postsynaptic neurons to presynaptic stimulation is restricted to the stimulated pathway. Post-tetanic potentiation is thus restricted to the particular afferent input channel over which stimulation is delivered. Whenever responses to stimulation change as a result of activity in one afferent pathway, but remain unchanged in response to activity in other afferent pathways, the process is termed "homosynaptic." Conversely, where activity in one afferent pathway can alter responses to other, nonstimulated pathways, the process is termed "heterosynaptic" (Kandel 1976). The prolongation of a high frequency stimulus may lead to changes, which persist for several hours in extreme cases.

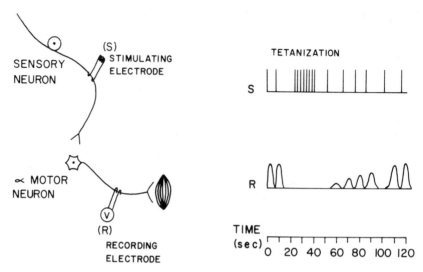

Figure 21.   Illustration of neural (action potential) patterning associated with post-tetanic potentiation.

The neural patterning associated with PTP is illustrated in Figure 21. The application of a standard test stimulus (S) elicits a moderate EPSP whose amplitude does not vary if the stimulus is repeated about 10 sec later. If a 20-sec period of tetanization occurs (between 20 and 40 sec), it is followed by enhanced EPSP responses to the standard test stimulus (facilitation) which may last beyond the period of rapid stimulation. During the 60 to 120 sec immediately after tetanization, the standard test stimulus evokes supranormal EPSP responses which gradually decay to normal levels.

After a period of brief tetanization, a subthreshold stimulus, which was previously incapable of eliciting action potentials in a postsynaptic neuron, may be capable of doing so as the result of PTP (Eccles 1953). Thus PTP increases the amplitude of response to both supra- and subthreshold stimulation and represents an elementary form of behavioral facilitation.

Post-tetanic depression (PTD) consists of repetitive high frequency stimulation of a neural pathway, resulting in a decrease in the number of postsynaptic or muscle cells responding to a stimulus as compared with responses to that stimulus seen before tetanization. Maximal depression usually occurs with periods of tetanization of about 30 sec. Longer periods of tetanization often result in facilitation. This phenomenon appears to be the opposite of PTP.

The patterning of action potentials associated with PTD is shown in Figure 22. Standard test stimuli (S) elicit standard amplitude responses (R) during the 0 to 15-sec period. Following tetanization of from 20 to 40 sec, a period of response amplitude depression occurs,

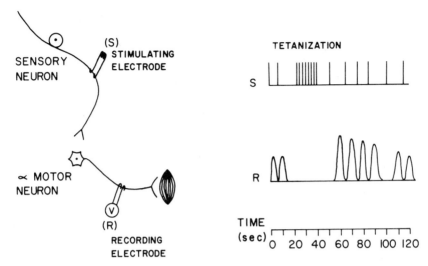

Figure 22.   Illustration of neural (action potential) patterning associated with post-tetanic depression.

after presentation of the standard test stimulus. This PTD lasts from 50 sec to about 120 sec and gradually returns to the pretetanization level of response.

Evarts and Hughes (1957) observed this form of cellular learning while recording from the lateral geniculate nucleus of the cat. When they tetanically stimulated the optic nerve at a rate of 500 times/sec, a profound depression of lateral geniculate activity resulted. Further study indicated that, unlike PTP which appears to endure longer if tetanization is longer, PTD was maximal when tetanic stimulation was close to 30 sec. Tetanic stimulation for much less than 30 sec was not as successful. Tetanic stimulation of more than 30 sec generally led to PTP rather than PTD (Kandel 1976).

A similarity between PTP and PTD is that both processes are homosynaptic, i.e., affect only stimulation presented via the tetanized pathway. The evidence concerning both PTP and PTD suggests an important principle of neural behavior: *There is apparently no simple relationship between either frequency of stimulation or length of time stimulated and the resulting changes in behavior that are observed.* Rapid stimulation may produce either augmentation or depression of responses. In certain pathways where potentiation occurs, an increase in stimulation time enhances the period of poststimulation retention of behavior changes, but where depression occurs, this is not the case. Changes in cellular or overt behavior cannot be predicted accurately from the frequency and/or duration of stimuli, nor is it possible to state that PTP leads to an increased behavioral response or PTD to a decreased response. Dudel and Kuffler (1961) and Waziri and colleagues (1969) have shown that PTP exists at synapses where the neurotransmitter is inhibitory as well as at those (such as the neuromuscular junction) where the neurotransmitter is excitatory. According to Woody (1982) the response of motor neurons to tetanic stimulation tends to be PTP at high frequencies and PTD at lower frequencies. At this time, the safest conclusion is that the behavioral responses of neurons to tetany is a function of tetanus length, frequency, strength, and specific neural membrane properties.

Learning serves adaptive purpose(s) and permits the individual to benefit from prior experiences. No clear-cut or definitive answer is possible to the question: What are the functions of PTP and PTD with respect to adaptation? Short-term learning paradigms (minutes to hours in duration) such as PTP and PTD have received relatively little consideration from psychologists and neurobiologists compared to intermediate and long-term learning.

Because the time for which behavior is modified by such learning is so brief, it might appear that PTP and PTD serve only transient adaptation. In this sense, they might act as fine-tuning on behavior to increase the efficiency of the neuromotor system's responses to high frequency stimulation. For example, at the neuromuscular junction where PTP has been demonstrated, its behavioral significance may be postulated. Any sustained voluntary muscular contraction in humans is the result of summed fusion of individual twitches rapidly following one another. Each efferent action potential may elicit a single twitch, but a volley or tetanizing pattern of action potentials is required for a smooth, sustained tetanic contraction.

Such tetanic contraction is the result of a high frequency volley of efferent action potentials from 10 to 50/sec. In fast glycolytic (pale) muscle fibers which show a very rapid rise to peak tension after a brief latency, the rate of efferent stimulation required for tetany is fairly high, perhaps 50-100 action potentials per second (Rasch and Burke 1974). Therefore, it can be speculated that during sustained voluntary muscular contraction, the role of PTP is to require fewer efferent action potentials to elicit successive voluntary contractions, in that each individual stimulus in the next voluntary chain of efferent action potentials will elicit an augmented or facilitated response. Hence, muscular tetany can be achieved with lower action potential frequencies than was possible before the first sustained contraction. Herein lies a quite plausible, albeit speculative, explanation of the value of warm-up before exertion. It might also explain that feeling of increased ease of voluntary effort after one or two initial repetitions. People say that they "find their groove" or "catch on" to the activity. In an event, the *neural demands* of a repeated muscular effort are less than those of the initial effort due to the effect of PTP. Post-tetanic potentiation at the neuromuscular junction is a short-lived phenomenon (usually for several minutes or less) that may increase the neural efficiency of voluntary activity and shorten the total time required to do a fixed amount of work by effectively "priming" muscles for repeated voluntary contraction.

Inasmuch as PTD has not been reported at the neuromuscular junction, it is difficult to comment on its role in adaptation. However, the longevity or brevity of PTP and PTD after initial learning is significant. These learning paradigms represent very short-term behavioral changes which permit the neural control of behavior to be enhanced or depressed for short periods as needed, but do not permanently alter the base response levels of the individual. The significance of such learning for therapeutic intervention, discussed in the next chapter, may shed light on the adaptive role of these short-term learning phenomena.

Habituation consists of a reversible decrease in the amplitude (strength) of a response when the response is repeatedly elicited through stimulation. A sudden or strong stimulus often restores immediately the original strength of the habituated response. This restoration is called "dishabituation," and is actually a form of sensitization—the learning paradigm to be considered next.

Unlike the short-term learning paradigms just discussed, habituation is universally accepted as worthy of consideration as a learning phenomenon (Kupferman 1975). All animals, including man, demonstrate this type of behavior modification (Kandel 1979c, 1979d).

In Figure 23A, the neural pattern associated with habituation is illustrated. With repeated applications of a standard non-noxious, low intensity stimulus (S_H) there is a gradual decline of response (R) amplitude on successive trials. Eventually the habituation stimulus fails to elicit any overt response, as shown in Trial 25.

Thorpe (1963) defined habituation as ". . . the relatively permanent waning of a response as a result of repeated stimulation which is not followed by any kind of reinforcement. It is specific to the stimulation and relatively enduring." Perhaps the most distinguishing characteristic of habituation is spontaneous recovery of habituated responses during periods of nonstimulation. Furthermore, the greater the period of nonstimulation, the more complete will be the recovery of the habituated response. Indeed, the degree of recovery of a response during a fixed time interval is a most useful measure of the strength of habituation, i.e., the less the recovery per unit time, the stronger the habituation (Petrinovich and Patterson 1979).

Bruner and Kennedy (1970) have applied an additional standard to define habituation operationally. They insist that any change in the frequency of stimulation, regardless of direction, will restore some of the habituated response. Others (Petrinovich and Patterson 1979) note that in addition to each of the above criteria, any novel stimulus

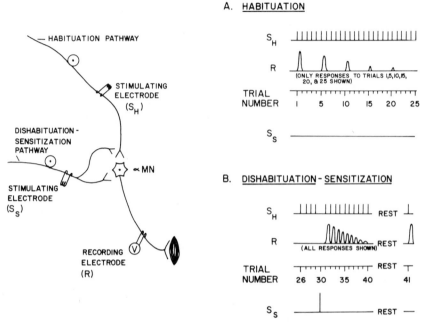

Figure 23.   *A:* The neural pattern associated with habituation and *B:* The neural pattern associated with sensitization (dishabituation).

or stimulus of significantly greater intensity (higher amplitude) leads to some degree of recovery of habituated responses. It is argued that this criterion is essential to rule out such phenomena as receptor adaptation and fatigue. This reversal of habituation by other strong or novel stimuli is referred to by the term "dishabituation," cited earlier.

The most comprehensive description of habituation is that of Thompson and Spencer (1966) and Thompson (1976). They report that the greater the number of habituation trials, the more complete the response depression. If the habituation stimulus is presented in a series of trials, the briefer the time interval between trials, the greater (and of course faster) the response depression. In other words, for a fixed number of habituation trials, the closer they are spaced in time, the more profound is the response decrement. There is also a relationship between stimulation intensity and rate of habituation. Given identical frequencies of stimulation, the weaker of two habituation stimuli virtually always produces the more rapid, complete habituations. This is to be expected because the weaker the initial stimulus, the weaker the response it elicits. Weak responses naturally require a smaller amplitude decline to reach a point of extinction. Finally, although habituated responses are capable of showing some degree of stimulus generalization (i.e., decreased responsiveness to stimuli similar to the habituation stimulus), for the most part, learning is restricted to the specific stimulus used to habituate that response.

Habituation is considered intermediate-term learning with respect to how long its effects endure. In many instances, the effects of repeated, non-noxious, and low-intensity stimulation last from several hours to several days. It has been reported that habituation may last 3-4 weeks after several sessions of 10 stimuli each (Kandel 1979b).

Little debate or doubt exists about the adaptive significance of this type of learning. Habituation functions to screen out information that has little immediate significance to the organism. Those environmental stimuli which occur repeatedly yet offer no threat to an individual usually are ignored because they do not signal a need for an adaptive response. For example, if you are working with a patient and another therapist begins a conversation nearby, you will glance that way to see what is going on. As the conversation continues, you will "forget" or ignore those sounds which were initially a distraction and focus solely on your patient. This decrease in your response (glancing and listening) with repeated stimulation is habituation. In fact, if the same process occurs the next day, you will again show an initial orientation response to the distracting stimuli, but habituation will be rapid. The period of "rest" from one day to the next is all that is required to restore your initial sensitivity.

There are three distinct adaptive functions performed by habituation. First, habituation serves to limit defensive and escape behaviors to those stimuli most likely to signal true danger. Any low intensity stimulus that poses little threat leads to rapid habituation of orienting and attending. Presumably, once free from the need to attend to each and every stimulus of the environment, only *novel* stimuli (be they dangerous or hedonic), elicit orientation and attending behaviors. Second, habituation helps the individual of a species to establish a territory. When the features of an environment are familiar, habituation occurs and decreases the need for exploratory and/or defensive behaviors. Presumably this permits attention and energy to be focused on appetitive and reproductive behaviors which enhance both individual and species survival. Finally, habituation serves a social function. Kinship bonds are maintained and strengthened by familiarity. Social behaviors seen and felt every day are acceptable and demand no special responses because habituation has dampened such tendencies. Deviant behavior, because it is not the norm and occurs infrequently, is met by attention, defensive behaviors, and responses designed to restore the status quo and suppress deviant behavior.

The functions of habituation cited thus far appear to be both simple and direct. There are also more complex functions of habituation.

One such example, that habituation may play a vital role in the neo-natal and early cognitive development of the child, has been pro-posed by Jeffrey (1968). The newborn child appears to orient toward and attend to virtually every stimulus in the environment. Because almost all stimuli are novel to the newborn and because most responses are initially reflexive, the infant appears to be motorically and perceptually "driven" by immediate surroundings. This does not mean that the infant is purely a stimulus-response organism whose behavior is wholly the result of environmental stimuli. As the newborn actively explores the environment, many novel stimuli will be encountered, some of which will have greater attraction and/or meaning for the infant than will others. Of course, even the newborn cannot attend to every stimulus. Certain more salient or powerful stimuli command attention and other less salient cues are ignored. As those perceptual features of the environment that are initially most important (e.g., mother's face, odor, body heat) are gradually habitu-ated, other cues, which might have initially been less relevant (toys, mobiles, etc.) may come to be powerful in commanding orienting and exploratory responses. In this manner, habituation serves to establish a hierarchy of attending responses that structure the sequence of perceptual learning. This serial habituation allows the infant to respond progressively to more subtle and complex features of the environment. Presumably, habituation enables the individual to focus and attend to relevant cues long enough to respond with behav-iors that maximize knowledge about the sources of these stimuli. Once these stimuli are familiar and demand no further exploratory responses (i.e., such responses have habituated), then other stimuli provoke exploration and attention. An illustration of this develop-mental role of habituation may be helpful. Take a 2-year-old child and a 15-year-old, and give each of them a large cardboard box. Say noth-ing to them, but observe their behavior. Chances are, the 15-year-old will look at the box, pick it up, look inside, and soon put it down. This is not likely to happen with the 2-year-old—the sequence of behavior will be highly variable but might include climbing onto or into the box, pulling and pushing it, banging on it, and perhaps tasting it. Because the 15-year-old has seen many other boxes like this one and has habituated effectively to the stimulus offered, the box holds little to excite or motivate exploration. For the 2-year-old, this box may engage attention and behavior for a considerable period of time.

It does not seem unreasonable to suppose that the "toys" of child-hood engage and fascinate because they teach the child about unfa-miliar features of the physical and symbolic world. Likewise, the same toys, familiar to an adult, would offer little that had not been repeatedly habituated. Developmentally, serial habituation keeps us exploring and manipulating objects until they are thoroughly familiar in most, if not all, respects. It also permits new objects, persons, and places to command attention so that they too may be explored. In complex series, these events contribute to the formation of stores of information about the world that are increasingly complex and diversified. This intermediate-term learning may serve both higher and more complex forms of learning by selectively focusing attention and by sequentially structuring perception of the environment.

Sensitization consists of an increase in the amplitude (strength) of a response to a given stimulus as a result of the presentation of another (often noxious or very strong stimulus) where such enhancement does not depend on pairing of the stimuli.

In its most general features sensitization is commonly regarded as the opposite of habituation as a form of learning. It is fundamentally a process whereby stimuli that predict either danger or significant novelty in the environment act to increase pre-existing reflexive behaviors (Kupferman 1975).

In Figure 23B, the neural pattern related to sensitization (dishabituation is *one* form of sensitization) is presented. Continued application of a habituation stimulus (S_H) beyond the point of zero amplitude response to a stimulus is shown in Trials 26–29. Not one of these four stimulus applications elicits a response (R). If on Trial 30, rather than applying a habituation stimulus (S_H), we apply a strong (high amplitude) novel stimulus over a sensitization pathway (S_S) it inevitably restores the habituated response to its original amplitude (Trial 31 in Fig. 23B above). This single strong stimulus totally reverses the effects of previous habituation learning. Trials 31–40 illustrate that if habituation is attempted after sensitization, it once again will lead to response decrements. Inasmuch as this is the repetition of habituation trials done earlier, it can also be seen that fewer trials of the habituation stimulus (S_H) are required to totally suppress the response. A period of rest after habituation also leads to a result similar to sensitization in that the original response is restored to its base line amplitude.

Sensitization can endure from minutes to weeks or longer after stimulation (Brunelli et al. 1976). This time course of sustained behavioral change is comparable to that of habituation and is the reason sensitization can be regarded as an intermediate-term learning paradigm.

Habituation shows only a very modest *stimulus* generalization. Sensitization, however, is highly generalized to *responses* other than those previously habituated. Greenbaum (1979) has pointed out that sensitization may be a critical component of behavioral arousal. Sensitization is a *heterosynaptic* phenomenon. That is, one in which activity in one input pathway influences and modifies activity in other input pathways, as well as modifying an output or response. In this respect, sensitization is more complex than habituation and resembles classical conditioning, with the notable exception that temporal pairing of stimuli is not necessary for sensitization but is necessary for classical conditioning (Castellucci and Kandel 1976).

The most widely studied form of sensitization was termed dishabituation for many years until it was recognized to be a process antagonistic to habituation, rather than an essential feature of habituation (Thompson and Spencer 1966). Sensitization has been found to be a powerful restorative force with respect to both very brief and very long habituated responses (Kandel 1979B).

The adaptive significance of sensitization can be considered both in its own right and with respect to habituation. Sensitization enables an individual to mobilize a range of responses to a single novel or threatening stimulus. Most of us have experienced a loud noise (such as a scream, explosion, or siren) interrupting our preoccupation with daily routines. Suddenly we are alert, eyes wide open, ears attentive, and heart racing! This sudden arousal is different from the response to an acquaintance who might interrupt us, but not startle us. In fact the word "acquaintance" connotes familiarity with the voice, appearance, and other "stimuli" of someone whom we have learned (via habituation and otherwise) poses no threat to us.

When sensitized by a scream or siren it is unusual to immediately return to one's previous occupation, and there is a heightening of responsiveness to most other stimuli, even nonthreatening ones. Not only is sensitization significant in its own right as a form of arousal, but it also serves to restore habituated responses to nonthreatening and familiar stimuli. One familiar example might be responses to household furnishings after sensitization from a sound during the night. We jump out of bed, turn on the lights, and immediately all of the familiar objects, furniture, doorways, and halls, elicit responses of attending and exploring even though no further sign of threat is present. For a period of time we have heightened arousal to all features of our environment. When a threat is present such dishabituation renders us cautious to *all* environmental features.

Sensitization, like habituation, serves to predict which classes of responses will be most appropriate in a given environment at a given time. Habituation predicts that failure to attend or respond to a given stimulus will be of little or no consequence. Sensitization predicts that failure to respond to even seemingly trivial stimuli could have dire consequences.

Classical conditioning is a process of repeatedly pairing a neutral stimulus with a stimulus that invariably elicits a response until the neutral stimulus alone is capable of eliciting the response (or one which closely resembles it). This type of learning is said to be "associative." The conditioned stimulus (CS) comes to be associated with (i.e., predicts) the unconditioned stimulus (UCS). This is the result of the close temporal association of these two stimuli. The CS also becomes associated with certain aspects or components of the response elicited by the UCS. During the period of training, stimuli are repeatedly paired with one another in an invariant sequence in which the CS always precedes the UCS and hence comes to predict that the UCS will follow whenever the CS is presented. The most widely noted example of classical conditioning was provided by Pavlov (1906) who observed that dogs salivated when their attendants appeared. In a series of experiments he presented a CS (bell) immediately before a UCS (food) and found that salivation, which always occurred reflexively to food presentation as part of an unconditioned response (UCR), would eventually occur as a conditioned response (CR) to the bell alone. The probable pattern of neural events associated with such learning is illustrated in Figure 24. During the pretest phase each presentation of UCS is represented here as a single spike for each stimulus (it could actually require more than a single spike to elicit the response). Presentations of the CS alone fail to elicit any responses.

Looking next at the training or acquisition phase, which typically consists of many more trials than shown in this illustration, each presentation of the CS is followed immediately by presentation of the UCS. The response (R) that results from each paired stimulus presentation is assumed to be the direct result of the UCS early in training because the CS is incapable of eliciting this response. Later in training the CS may come to be associated as a prediction of the UCS and may begin to influence responses. Finally, during the post-training period the results of associative classical conditioning are illustrated in that the CS or UCS, when presented alone, are each capable of eliciting the response that originally could be obtained only by UCS presentation.

One interpretation of the classical conditioning process is that the associative learning that occurs is critically dependent on the specific temporal ordering of training events. Such an interpretation implies that behavior changes because the individual is able to reliably predict that a neutral stimulus (CS) will be followed by a UCS (Walters et al. 1979). It is generally accepted that the optimal ordering of events for classical conditioning is to have the CS precede the UCS (Munsinger 1975). Furthermore, the optimal interval between CS and UCS is generally accepted to be from one-half second to several seconds (Logue 1979). The one notable exception to the general principle that optimal conditioning requires very brief delays is taste-aversion learning whereby consuming a food (CS) that leads to gastric distress (UCS) resulting in vomiting and/or nausea (R) leads to effective learned aversion even if the delay interval between stimuli is quite long (Logue 1979).

Classical conditioning can be classified into two broad categories

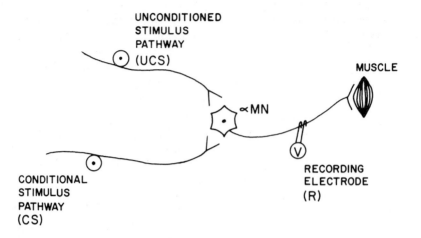

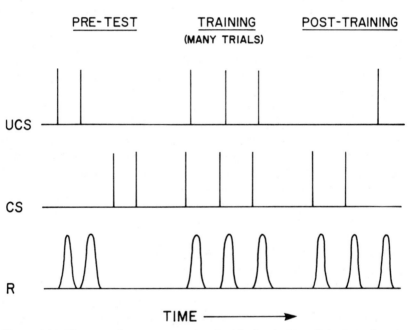

Figure 24.   The neural pattern associated with classical conditioning wherein a neutral stimulus (CS) is paired with an unconditional stimulus (UCS) to elicit a response (R) even when the UCS is not presented.

based on the nature of the UCS. Whenever the UCS is pleasurable or rewarding the association of CS with the UCS is termed appetitive conditioning and consumatory or approach behavior is generally the R to such stimulation. When the UCS is either noxious or punitive and the resulting R consists of either protective or escape (avoidance) behaviors, then the conditioned association of a neutral CS with such UCS is termed defensive conditioning (Kupferman 1981).

Reversal of learning, or extinction, is an important feature of classical conditioning. If a CR has been repeatedly elicited by a CS in the absence of any UCS presentations, then over time the intensity of the CR or the likelihood of its occurring after CS presentation will decrease.

This is quite similar to the "forgetting" of habituated responses which follows a period of nonstimulation. In the case of classical conditioning this phenomenon is known as extinction. Its adaptive significance seems to be that it eliminates from an individual's repertoire those conditioned responses that no longer predict an association between two stimuli. Kupferman (1981) has further observed that extinction is most likely due to active processes rather than to a passive reversal of changes serving the learned behavior.

Although classical conditioning can be extinguished, it is appropriately considered to be long-term learning. In some cases of both appetitive and defensive conditioning a period of training may be sufficient to establish a CS-associated response that lasts the lifetime of the individual. Such learning is said to be relatively resistant to extinction. It is important to recognize that many forms of classical conditioning represent learning in relation to stimuli that are naturally paired. Where such natural pairing exists "training" is inherent in an individual's experience. Food preferences are an example of such natural learned associations. A person sees and smells food (both CS) before experiencing the taste (UCS) which leads to a response (R_1) of salivation, mastication, and swallowing and more importantly to a response (R_2) of obtaining more of the same food. We naturally continue to select and eat (R_2) foods which look and smell (CS_S) as if they will taste good (UCS).

The adaptive significance of classically conditioned learning has been discussed and explored by many learning theorists. For the purpose of this discussion it is not feasible to explore all possible adaptive advantages of classical conditioning, but only the more obvious contributions to adaptation which are served by such learning.

Classical conditioning is established in human infants within 3–4 days after birth (Munsinger 1975). Of what value is such learning so early in life?

Mother-infant bonding has received considerable attention in recent years. One issue is to determine the degree to which common maternal-infant experiences influence such bonding. Freud suggested that infants sought close contact with their mothers because of the pleasurable (appetitive) association of the mother (CS) with the taste of her milk (UCS) and the visceral responses (UCR) elicited by the milk. Recent studies with infant rats, in which neutral olfactory stimuli (CS) were paired with milk (UCS) or no milk delivery while sucking a passive dam, showed that rat pups acquired a significantly greater preference for those odors paired with milk presentation over those paired with no milk (Brake 1981). Although the extrapolation of results from rats to humans can be justifiably questioned, the study represents the first evidence that milk delivery in mammals may be responsible for developing learned associations between maternal behavior and infant responses. Replication of this study using human subjects is clearly indicated.

Defensive classical conditioning appears to serve both adaptive and maladaptive behavioral learning. One form of learning, called rapid aversive conditioning, takes advantage of innate defensive and/or escape responses. Thus a neutral stimulus (CS) such as the visual image of a dog, if followed by a painful scratch or bite (UCS) to a child, may appropriately lead to avoiding other dogs by running away, screaming, or hiding (all UCRs and CRs). It appears that rapid learning such as this is facilitated or "prepared" insofar as the CRs, such as putting the hands in front of the face or freezing, are natural defensive reactions (Logue 1979).

Many fears appear to be the result of classically associated stimuli. During the period of toilet training, a young child may come to associate the neutral stimulus of the bathroom with feelings of inadequacy or failure (mother criticizes or scolds child), and thus develop a conditional fear of bathrooms (Munsinger 1975). The pervasiveness of such conditioning is attested to by Kushner (1981): "How many public and private superstitions are based upon something good or bad happening right after we did something, and our assuming that the same thing will follow the same pattern every time?"

By far the most dramatic example of classical conditioning is the association of "neutral" symbols, especially words, with emotional events. "Love" is wonderful only as the result of being held (UCS), caressed (UCS), kissed (UCS), and smiled at (UCS). The expression, "I love you," derives its power from previous paired associations of action-oriented stimuli with the utterance of the symbolic statement. Imagine saying, "I love you," over the phone to someone who speaks no English. The auditory stimulus itself is truly neutral! What "love" is differs from person to person, in part because the associations of events differ with the word "love." For most people, words eventually come to have a power of their own. It takes a rational mind to recognize that someone saying you are a "no good, worthless, despicable slob" neither makes us *be* that, nor does it make us *feel* bad about being called such names. Rather, we are simply victims of our prior learned associations.

Why do emotionally laden terms seem especially susceptible to such associations? Perhaps because other more neutral terms such as "brown-haired" or "carpenter" are not likely to have occurred under conditions in which visceral or affective sensations (UCSs) were present and gave rise to automatic or stereotyped responses (UCRs).

Thus, for words that are rarely paired with situations having high affective content (good or bad) the likelihood of classically conditioned verbal associations is decreased. It is not only what we say but how we say it that determines meaning. If one says "I love you" with a sarcastic or nasty tone the message received will not be interpreted as an expression of genuine affection.

Each of the examples cited thus far focuses on some autonomic or visceral response. By and large, there has been a tendency to identify classical conditioning with autonomic response learning and instrumental conditioning with skeletal movements learning. Such a view may accurately reflect a general tendency but ignores ever-increasing evidence that both types of conditioning have been employed to train autonomic and somatic motor learning (Hearst 1975).

It is necessary to place the study of classical conditioning in a reasonable perspective. First, most traditional classical conditioning studies have focused on the stimulus events and qualities while ignoring any measures of response events other than frequency of UCRs and CRs. As Martin and Levey (1969) have noted, "This is about as useful an analysis of conditioning as a count of key presses is of a pianist's performance." The effects of stimulus intensity, frequency, CS-UCS delay length, and stimulus significance have received inordinate emphasis compared to studies of response latency, response amplitude, and variability of responses during conditioning. Second, it is often assumed that classical conditioning is highly specific, i.e., a single reflexive response is brought under control of a neutral stimulus. Moreover, autonomic or visceral activity (e.g., salivation, galvanic skin response, and such) has generally been used as the response events. Schwartz et al. (1971) reviewed the literature on conditioned learning and concluded:

> . . . both autonomic and skeletal movements of the whole organism can be conditioned via *either* classical conditioning *or* instrumental conditioning procedures.

and

> . . . a pattern of functionally related behaviors, not a single response is being conditioned in any classical or operant conditioning experiment. The artificial restrictions of the laboratory environment have misled many researchers into a false assumption that other behaviors (not measured during the experiment), were not altered during the course of learning.

Instrumental or operant conditioning consists of the presentation of a reinforcing stimulus after the occurrence of a given response so that repeated presentations of the reinforcing stimulus lead to an increase in the frequency and/or probability of the reinforced response.

Just as classical conditioning is said to be associative, so too is instrumental conditioning. Classical conditioning procedures create an association of two stimuli, the unconditional stimulus which reflexively evokes responses and the conditional stimulus which initially does not elicit such responses but comes to do so after careful pairing or temporal association with the UCS. Instrumental or operant conditioning procedures create an association not between two stimuli, but between a response and a stimulus that follows. Kupferman (1981:570–573) notes that, "Unlike classical conditioning, which is restricted to specific reflex responses that are evoked by specific, identifiable stimuli, operant conditioning involves behaviors (called operants) that apparently occur spontaneously or with no recognizable eliciting stimuli."

Instrumental conditioning may be used to modify behaviors which are, in contrast to classically conditioned responses, appropriately termed "emitted" behaviors (operants). These are modified by the presentation of reinforcing stimuli following the occurrence of the behavior. Since such behaviors often have no clear link to prior stimuli, they are most often considered "voluntary" behaviors.

Associative learning paradigms take great care to distinguish between classes of stimulus events. Two such classes have already been described: *eliciting stimuli,* which call forth a reflexive response, and *reinforcing stimuli,* which follow as consequences of voluntary or spontaneous behaviors. Stimuli act to set the stage or signal conditions that are ideal for behaviors reinforced previously (Brady 1979).

Two distinct classes of behaviors also are influenced by associative learning paradigms: *reflexive responses* or *respondents,* which usually occur after eliciting stimuli, and operants or *voluntary responses,* whose frequency is modified by reinforcing stimuli.

Instrumental conditioning was described first by Thorndike (1898) as the "law of effect," which proposed that rewards or reinforcing stimuli served to connect responses to stimuli and that large rewards produce stronger associations than small rewards. In other words, behaviors that produce the greatest pleasurable or hedonic consequences are established more reliably than those which produce the least pleasurable consequences (Bitterman 1975).

Just as Pavlov above all others is identified with classical conditioning, Skinner's (1938, 1965) name is most often associated with instrumental conditioning. Skinner's contribution was to focus on the modification of virtually any and all voluntary behaviors through the selective use of rewards and punishments.

The pattern of neural events associated with instrumental conditioning is illustrated in Figure 25. During the pretest phase, the behavior that is to be modified occurs voluntarily (or otherwise) at some frequency that can be expressed as the number of occurrences per unit of time. This behavior is the response shown twice during

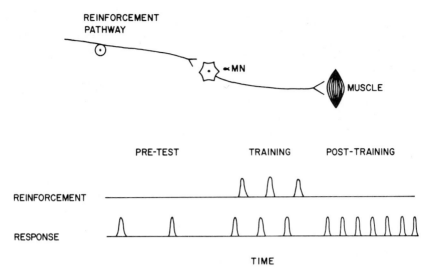

Figure 25. The neural pattern associated with instrumental or operant conditioning wherein a stimulus reinforcement which follows an emitted response will subsequently alter the frequency of that response.

the pretest phase in Figure 25. Note that no eliciting or reinforcing stimulus is presented before or after this response. During training, the response again occurs naturally, only now it is followed by a reinforcement or reward stimulus. Although there are many different "schedules" of reinforcement that may be effective, only the simplest example—that of continuous reinforcement—is shown here. Repeated reinforcement of responses increases the frequency of the response during training making it greater than during the pretest. Finally, during the post-training periods, even if no reinforcement is provided, response frequency will increase over the pretest frequency. If reinforcement is totally ceased after training, a gradual decline in the "learned" frequency change will occur, and such non-reinforcement is said to lead to the *extinction* of the learned component of behavior.

Reinforcing stimuli fall into one of three primary classes. They are either positive reinforcers, which are rewards, or negative reinforcers, which consist of the removal or avoidance of aversive stimuli, or punishments, which are noxious stimuli. A common misconception is that positive reinforcers increase and punishment decreases the frequency of operants. Actually, under the right circumstances, rewards can be used to extinguish behaviors and punishments used to increase the frequency of behavior. To understand this it is necessary to consider the motivation of an individual to respond with a given behavior. White (1959) provides extensive evidence for at least three different types of motivation. He calls such motivations "drives." First are the primary drives, which represent conditions such as hunger and thirst and are associated with tissue deficits. They exist in a similar fashion for all members of a species. Behaviors such as *searching* for food and/or water, *increase* with nonreinforcement but actually *decrease* with any positive reinforcement or reward that reduces the tissue deficit (e.g., food or water). Punishment of such behaviors only temporarily decreases frequency of searching behavior and withdrawal of such punishment leads to increases in behaviors that seek to satisfy the need for food and water.

Next come secondary "drives." These may be thought of as hedonic drives in contrast to primary drives which are distinctly "survival" oriented. Secondary drives include desires for recognition or approval, desires for money, and desires for certain objects such as cars, stereos, etc. Note that secondary drives are often called "desires" whereas primary drives are called "needs." Behaviors such as working at a task to gain recognition increase in frequency when positively reinforced and decrease in frequency when nonreinforced or punished. For secondary drives, the association of positive reinforcement with increased operant frequency and punishment with decreased operant frequency is most appropriate.

Finally, there are drives that do not clearly fall into either of the above categories. White calls these "competence drives"; they include the need to manipulate objects, to explore one's environment, and to move one's body from place to place within one's environment. Although positive reinforcement tends to increase such behaviors and punishment to decrease them, there appear to be certain minimal "needs" for such activity. Thus, if all movement, manipulation, and exploration are nonreinforced or even punished, the behaviors tend to increase in frequency. (For example, try punishing a child for not sitting still, i.e., squirming in a chair.) On the other hand, positive reinforcement most often increases behaviors that tend to fulfill competency "needs."

To predict the effects of a given reinforcer, one must know something about the individual's motivation to perform an act and what has gone on previously with that individual and the environment. It is hoped that the misconception that rewards always increase frequency of behavior and negative reinforcement decreases frequency of behavior will be replaced by a more accurate understanding of motivational influences. Another issue centers on which behavior is the operant one desires to modify? For example, if one places a rat in a cage with a metal strip dividing the cage into two parts and wishes to have the rat leap from one side to the other across the plate, it is easier to obtain that behavior by punishing walking across the grid (i.e., by electrifying the metal strip so that it shocks the rat if touched) than it is to positively reward the highly improbable event that the rat will decide to jump over the strip, rather than walk across it.

Apropos of punishment, it should be noted that punishment suppresses but does not extinguish operants. Behaviors usually revert to pretraining levels once the punishment is removed. Furthermore punishment has been found to usually elicit unpredictable responses from its victims (Woody 1982). Only with intense punishment is it common to suppress an undesirable behavior. In general, nonreinforcement (ignoring) is a more effective means of extinguishing behaviors than is punishment.

If instrumental conditioning only alters the frequency of an emitted response, one might wonder how the individual can learn new behaviors. That this is possible seems self-evident. Let's take sewing as an example. Not one of us was born knowing how to sew. It is also highly improbable that sewing is a series of classically conditioned reflexes which we have learned through stimulus—stimulus associations. How then did we learn to sew? (For the reader who doesn't sew, substitute some other act such as feeding oneself.)

The instrumental process whereby such complex learning occurs is known as *shaping* or *successive approximations*. Brady (1979:26) provides an excellent description of this phenomenon:

> . . . it has been possible to make explicit the process called *shaping*, whereby a combination of operant conditioning and *extinction* (i.e., withholding reinforcers) can shape existing simple responses into new and more complex performances. Of critical importance for this shaping process is the observation that a reinforcing stimulus not only strengthens the particular response that precedes it, but also results in an increase in the frequency of many other bits of behavior (i.e., *response generalization*) and in effect raises the individual's general activity level.
>
> Thus, the shaping of behavior proceeds, as reinforcers are initially presented following a response similar to or approximating the desired one. Since this tends to increase the strength of various other similar behaviors, a response still closer to the desired can be selected from this new array and followed by reinforcing stimuli. Continued narrowing and refinement of the response criteria required for reinforcement leads progressively to new arrays of available behavior. . . . This shaping process is obviously of enormous clinical importance in behavioral medicine since many patient performances can only be changed effectively in this way.

Operant conditioning is long-term learning. It may endure months, years, even the lifetime of an individual. The retention of such learning clearly depends on memory, which is a subject beyond the scope of this book. But the single most important determinant of longevity of learning is the *schedule of reinforcement* used to establish and maintain operant learning. A reinforcement schedule is a set of criteria or rules that state under which circumstances specifically defined reinforcement will be provided. It is impossible in most cases to know how much is being "forgotten" or lost and when such "forgetting" occurs. Longevity of learning is therefore not directly assessed.

Instead, we measure the *resistance to extinction* or the degree to which operant conditioned behavior is maintained even when no reinforcement is given.

One quality of reinforcement schedules is the nature of the reinforcer: positive, negative, nonreinforcement, or punishment. Another key dimension is timing. Often a reinforcer must follow soon after the operant behavior or conditioning will be decreased (Kupferman 1981). The extensive research on children generally shows that the best learning occurs when reinforcement is immediate (*see* Munsinger 1975 for examples).

When a reinforcement schedule requires every operant response to be reinforced (positively or negatively) the schedule is termed *continuous reinforcement*. When only certain occasions of operant responding are reinforced, then the schedule is termed *partial reinforcement*. A major principle of operant conditioning is that resistance to extinction is greater using schedules of partial reinforcement than it is using schedules of continuous reinforcement. For example, if we continuously praise a patient for every small component of performance, we may be less successful in altering behavior than when we wisely praise only significant and/or new accomplishments. Continuous reinforcement may cause an individual to *habituate* to the reinforcing stimulus and therefore its effect may be diminished. Since continuous reinforcement schedules are rarely appropriate, it is best to focus on partial reinforcement schedules. These fall into two broad categories each of which can be subdivided into two primary subcategories as shown in Figure 26. The major categories are *ratio* and *interval* reinforcement and the subcategories of each are *fixed* or *variable* patterns of reinforcement (Brady 1979).

Ratio reinforcement schedules are those that stipulate how many *times* an operant behavior must occur before it is reinforced. If reinforcements are provided at ratios that approach continuous reinforcement, the risk of decreased retention occurs. On the other hand, if an individual is only rewarded after many expressions of an operant behavior, there is a danger of extinction occurring during training because the behavior desired is not reinforced much of the time.

Interval reinforcement schedules provide for reinforcement at specified time intervals during performance, independent of how many times the operant behavior has occurred. Interval schedules can also approach or even surpass continuous reinforcement if the intervals are too brief. Likewise, if intervals are too long, extinction will occur during training. But unlike ratio schedules, interval schedules have built-in reinforcement for persisting at a task even if the target behavior occurs only rarely. Where a ratio schedule would discourage a slow learner or one in the early stages of learning, an interval schedule essentially rewards trying to learn.

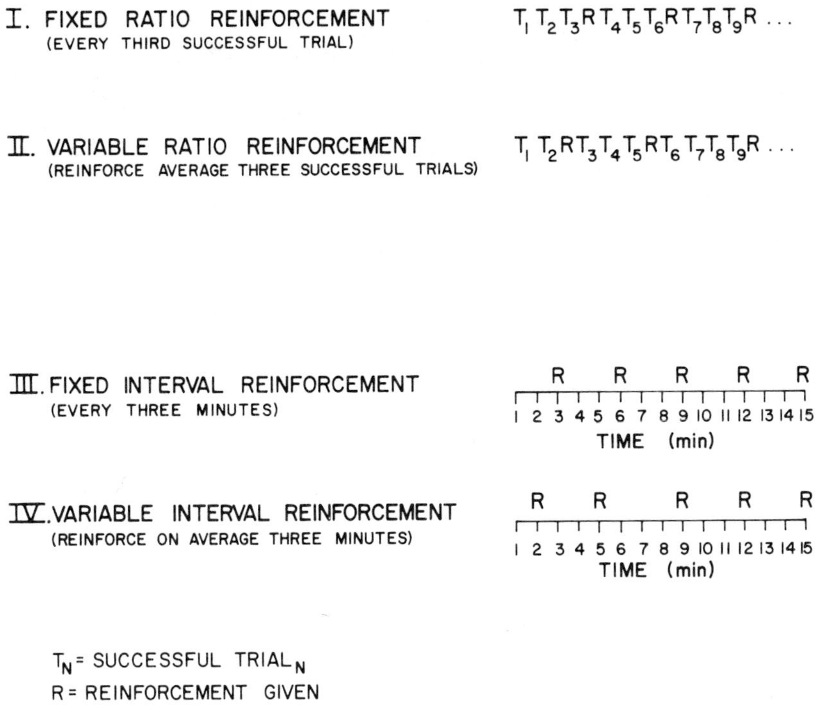

I. FIXED RATIO REINFORCEMENT
(EVERY THIRD SUCCESSFUL TRIAL)

$T_1 \, T_2 \, T_3 R \, T_4 \, T_5 \, T_6 R \, T_7 \, T_8 \, T_9 R \cdots$

II. VARIABLE RATIO REINFORCEMENT
(REINFORCE AVERAGE THREE SUCCESSFUL TRIALS)

$T_1 \, T_2 R T_3 \, T_4 \, T_5 R T_6 \, T_7 \, T_8 \, T_9 R \cdots$

III. FIXED INTERVAL REINFORCEMENT
(EVERY THREE MINUTES)

```
     R      R      R      R      R
  |--|--|--|--|--|--|--|--|--|--|--|--|--|--|--|
  1  2  3  4  5  6  7  8  9 10 11 12 13 14 15
              TIME   (min)
```

IV. VARIABLE INTERVAL REINFORCEMENT
(REINFORCE ON AVERAGE THREE MINUTES)

```
  R         R          R       R         R
  |--|--|--|--|--|--|--|--|--|--|--|--|--|--|--|
  1  2  3  4  5  6  7  8  9 10 11 12 13 14 15
              TIME   (min)
```

T_N = SUCCESSFUL TRIAL$_N$
R = REINFORCEMENT GIVEN

Figure 26. Examples of reinforcement schedules in operant conditioning.

Ratio and interval schedules can be either *fixed*, i.e., the ratio or interval is constant, or *variable*, i.e., the ratio or intervals may change during training. With fixed schedules, the learner not only learns the operant behaviors desired but also learns the schedule, and performance is altered in anticipation of those conditions that determine when reinforcement will occur. With variable schedules, learning about the schedule itself is difficult or impossible, and the seemingly random nature of reinforcement tends to minimize strategies that seek to perform at different levels during training.

Using these four major types of reinforcement schedules, virtually every more complex schedule can be described. For example, a given behavior may be reinforced only if it meets the requirements of two or more schedules. This is termed a *compound schedule*. Or we may wish to provide reinforcement only if two or more behaviors (operants) meet the simultaneous demands of two or more reinforcement schedules. This is termed a *concurrent schedule*. Other complex schedules fall into the categories of *multiple schedules*. In most natural learning situations, reinforcement typically follows compound, concurrent, or complex schedules (Brady 1979). This is of great significance for therapists and will be elaborated upon in chapter 3. The key finding related to reinforcement schedules is that the rate and duration of operant learning can best be controlled through the careful design and implementation of schedules of reinforcement.

If this principle is related to the underlying neural events that serve operant conditioning, then it clearly supports the major premise of this chapter; namely that the *patterning* of action potentials (in which all stimuli and responses are expressed) is an important determinant of the nature and extent of learning.

Individual differences greatly influence operant conditioning. What is a reward for one person may not be so for another. Not only does drive level influence motivation and response to reinforcers but also age, social class, and previous exposure to reinforcers (Munsinger 1975). Any task for which we wish to shape or train behavior will have a hierarchy of positive and negative reinforcers. How rewards are selected and in what order makes a difference in outcome. Bitterman (1975) found that rats who were initially reinforced with a highly preferred reward performed significantly less well than untrained controls when a less-favored reward was used. Americans have recently seen many manifestations of this phenomenon related to salaries during an economic slump with high inflation. Rather than accept their same jobs with reduced pay (a lesser reward) many chose to take their chances on being laid off (greatly reduced rewards) and not compromise salary demands during collective bargaining negotiations. One may think of a weekly or monthly salary as a fixed interval schedule of reinforcement. Presumably, we learn that even though each individual effort we put forth will not be rewarded immediately, there will come a time when rewards will be received (Kupferman 1981).

Any attempt to appreciate the relationship between environmental events (stimuli) associated with operant conditioning and the underlying neural events must acknowledge the complexity of most reinforcing stimuli. A simple reward such as food has sensory components of vision, olfaction, gustation, and chemoreception all of which translate into action potentials. If any of these are unpleasant (i.e., punishment) such as food that looks appetizing but has an unpleasant odor, then the value as a reinforcement is compromised. In such a case, both positive and punishing reinforcers are received and the reward value is decreased. The complexity of multimodal stimuli is especially important with social reinforcers such as verbal approval, attention, privileges, and the like. For example, if I tell a burn victim that his disfigured face really looks pretty good then I must be certain to maintain eye contact and be aware that all of my nonverbal behaviors support my verbal statement. Indeed, when we say we give a person "mixed messages" what we are often doing is both rewarding and punishing the same behavior or asking simultaneously for behaviors that are mutually incompatible.

Such an analysis leads to what I term the "neural necessity" for *honesty* in therapy. Feedback to a patient that presents complex stimuli must be free of mixed positive and punitive reinforcers. Honest feedback is operant guidance that is clear and direct. If one is not honest it is possible to send mixed messages that will impede the course of therapeutic learning. Being honest need not imply that one tell each patient every detail concerning that person's condition. A therapist should always be careful not to deprive a patient of all hope.

Situations in which a therapist would *like* to give positive reinforcement but doesn't feel it is merited can tempt one to give reinforcement on an interval schedule to avoid having to wait for appropriate operant responses. This is certainly acceptable. But in many cases such conflicts tell the therapist that the failure is one of not appropriately *shaping* behavior. By rewarding successive approximations to the desired behavior such difficulties may be minimized.

Finally, do classical and instrumental conditioning truly represent distinct learning paradigms? There is ample evidence to suggest that both kinds of conditioning can be applied to either visceral or skeletal muscle responses (Hearst 1975). In both types of learning the temporal relationships of stimuli determine the extent of learning (Kupferman 1981). In considering the cellular mechanisms of the six paradigms of learning, we find that the neural mechanisms of both classical and instrumental learning may be the same. Given these statements, why do I choose to present classical and instrumental conditioning as distinct rather than as related types of learning? First, as noted, classical conditioning develops associations between *stimulus* and *stimulus*, whereas instrumental conditioning develops associations between *stimulus* consequences and *responses*. Second, classical conditioning deals with reflexive or elicited behaviors, whereas instrumental conditioning deals with "volitional" responses. Finally, although the cellular mechanisms may be similar or even the same, the patterns of action potentials related to learned changes in behavior are not the same for both classical and instrumental conditioning. For these reasons I consider learning using six paradigms rather than five. The reader should recall that this book presents a certain bias of viewpoint—one chosen for its utility to therapists—and well supported by both basic science and clinical evidence. Learning itself may be more complex than I suggest. As Kupferman (1981) notes:

> In addition to classical and operant conditioning there are other more complex types of learning. Although these higher forms of learning differ in detail from the simpler types we have considered, there is reason to believe that the broad principles of learning apply to many types of learning. At the same time, however, knowledge of the details of the specific learning tasks and of the capabilities of the individuals involved can make the difference between successful and unsuccessful application of learning principles to specific species of animals or to individual clinical cases.

The examination of each of the six paradigms of learning, both with respect to neural patterns associated with each and their behavioral significance, has been completed. Before progressing to the application of this conceptual framework to therapeutic intervention, information concerning the cellular correlates of learning is presented. This is the current focus of many neuroanatomists and neurophysiologists, and represents the development of a basic science of learning, so it is important to know something of recent developments in the cellular neurobiology of learning.

NEURAL MECHANISMS OF LEARNING

Our definition of learning as a change in behavior or responsiveness as a result of previous experiences (exposure to stimuli) is broad and all encompassing. Yet learning is not a single phenomenon. Kandel (1979a) has observed that ''. . . learning is not one process, but rather a family of processes, presumably involving a variety of cellular mechanisms. . . .'' To better understand how learning can occur at the cellular level one must review the properties of neurons. Buchtel and Berlucci (1977) suggest that there are two properties, *reactivity* and *plasticity*, that serve learning.

Reactivity of neurons has been discussed earlier in chapter 1. All neurons are excitable cells which respond to changes in environmental energy (stimuli). Such cells also transmit an electrical potential record of stimulus events along their own cell membranes and a chemical record across synapses to excite or inhibit other nerve cells. In addition to being responsible for mediating sensory, motor, and integrating events, neurons are capable of modifying their *own* reactivity via changes in their structure (morphology) and their functioning (physiology). Kornorski (1968) terms such modifications ''plasticity'' and describes them as alterations in structure and/or function as a result of previous activation. He emphasized strongly that ''plastic'' changes were different from those changes in structure or function of neurons due to growth, development, injury, or aging of neurons (*for review see* Buchtel and Berlucci 1977).

Unfortunately, this original concept of ''plasticity'' has been somewhat confused by a more general clinical definition of plasticity that includes either genetically preprogrammed ontogenic changes or the response and recovery from injury. Neurobiologists studying learning seem to prefer the original, and more restrictive, definition. The central tenet of this concept of plasticity is that all stimuli produce a time-dependent and a transient change in neural activity (reactivity), but that only certain specific stimulus patterns lead to alterations that create enduring functional changes in systems of neurons (Kandel 1981).

Are plastic changes in neural systems the result of stimulus-induced structural (morphological and/or biochemical) changes in neurons? Are they the result of changes in the physiologic strength of cellular or synaptic functions? Or does some combination of anatomic and physiologic mechanisms best explain learning at the cellular level? Although there are still no definitive answers to these questions, the preponderance of evidence over the past 10-15 years seems to suggest that plastic changes related to learning are best described as being due to functional modifications in synaptic transmission, which occur without significant changes in cell structure (Bruner and Kennedy 1970; Castellucci and Kandel 1976; Mpitsos et al. 1978; Walters et al. 1979; Carew et al. 1981; Woody 1982).

Buchtel and Berlucci (1977) summarize the current position of most neurobiologists of learning:

1. The general plan of the connections within the nervous system is laid out by heredity alone, but proper functioning of the connections must be maintained or brought out by interactions with the environment, especially during the maturation period.

2. Specific environmental influences resulting in learning act by modifying interneuronal communication at one or more of the synapses already existing in the connection system produced by heredity and maturation.

Those familiar with longstanding debate over "Nature vs. Nurture" as determinants of behavior will appreciate the profound implications of this position. Nature, through genetic expression, has specified the plan of connectedness within each nervous system, not only the general patterns but each neuron and perhaps each synapse. What these processes do not determine is the *strength* or *effectiveness* of each neuron and synapse. Nurture or environmental experiences, via processes we call learning, function to alter the strength of these connections depending on the individual's history of interactions with the environment.

The problems of studying the cellular mechanisms of learning deserve comment. The human nervous system consists of more than one trillion neurons. The number of possible connections between these is greater by far than the number of atoms in the entire universe! Human cellular studies also pose ethical issues that preclude such investigations (Kandel 1979b). Bitterman (1975) has reviewed the work of Pavlov, Thorndike, and many others and concludes that all behavioral evidence suggests that invertebrate and vertebrate nervous systems respond similarly to stimulation. Furthermore, each of the six paradigms of learning seem to be present in vertebrates and invertebrates, which suggests that common mechanisms may serve all species. The neurons of all species are amazingly similar in their behavior. This does not prove that cellular mechanisms described in animal preparations also apply to humans; nevertheless there are certainly reasons for tentatively extrapolating animal findings from one species to another.

Thompson and Spencer (1966) laid the foundations for much of today's research, which seeks to relate the cellular events of learning to the changes in behavior that occur. They suggested:

> Perhaps the most fundamental problem in physiological psychology is the elucidation of neuronal mechanisms underlying alterations in behavior. This implies prediction of behavioral changes from descriptions in terms of patterns of synaptic interactions among identifiable populations of neurons.

The ability to record the physiologic and biochemical activity of single neurons, using micropipette electrodes, has aided the identification of entire behaviors (feeding, swimming, withdrawal) of simple invertebrates, in which every neuron (motor, sensory, and interneuron) that served such behavior was identifiable and present in all members of the species. Such simple networks have enabled neurobiologists to study all six paradigms of learning in simple animals.

A guiding question of cellular studies of learning has been "How many kinds of learning are there?" There may be a distinct cellular mechanism for each learning paradigm, but it is also possible that a very few simple mechanisms could serve different behavioral changes. The options regarding mechanisms can be reduced to a relatively few anatomic sites. Plastic alterations serving learning occur either in presynaptic neurons or in postsynaptic neurons. (It may be that pre- and postsynaptic sites could both be altered, but I can find no evidence of this in my search of the literature.) Additionally, these changes may either be *homosynaptic*—i.e., restricted to the neurons directly stimulated during "learning"—or they may be *heterosynaptic*—i.e., affect neurons not directly stimulated but which can elicit the learned behaviors. Thus, there are four possible combinations to consider:

1. Presynaptic—homosynaptic site.
2. Presynaptic—heterosynaptic site.
3. Postsynaptic—homosynaptic site.
4. Postsynaptic—heterosynaptic site.

Kandel (1976) explains that:

> Increased effectiveness of synaptic transmission could be caused either by a presynaptic mechanism—an increase in the number of transmitter quanta released by the presynaptic terminals per unit impulse, or by a postsynaptic mechanism—an increased responsiveness of the postsynaptic receptor to a constant quantal output, or an increase in input resistance, or a decrease in threshold.

For each of the paradigms considered, it is now possible to identify sites at which plastic changes occur, and for some of the learning paradigms additional knowledge of mechanisms is available. Let us review each type of learning and illustrate briefly the progress being made at linking cellular activity to the behaviors that are served by such activity.

Kandel (1976, 1981) and Woody (1982) have thoroughly reviewed the cellular bases of learning. Those interested in reading the primary research literature on this subject will find extensive references in the reviews cited. Except where otherwise noted, the information presented below is extracted from Kandel or Woody:

Post-tetanic potentiation and post-tetanic depression were both found by Lloyd (1949) to be homosynaptic phenomena. Liley (1956) analyzed the mechanism of PTP in the rat nerve-muscle synapse. He found that the amplitude of the spontaneous miniature end plate potentials (*see* chapter 1) did not change as a result of PTP. Since unitary MEPPs represent the effects of a single quantum of neurotransmitter being released, a failure to find a change in MEPP amplitude clearly indicated that changes in postsynaptic sensitivity did not occur as a result of PTP. Consequently, Liley also showed that the average number of quanta of neurotransmitter released presynaptically increased during PTP. Rosenthal (1969) verified this at the frog neuromuscular junction. He also found, as had Katz and Miledi (1965), that PTP was due to increased accumulations of calcium in presynaptic terminals, which in turn resulted in increased probabilities of transmitter release. Unfortunately, evidence concerning the mechanisms of PTD is not as advanced as for PTP at the present time.

Habituation in aplysia, a sea-snail, has been found by Kandel (1981) and many others to involve a decrease in the ability of sensory neurons to elicit responses from their target cells. Recall that habituation may be thought of as learning to ignore stimuli that pose little or no threat to an organism. By measuring the EPSPs produced in motor cells by repetitive non-noxious stimulation, it has been found that each successive presynaptic action potential elicits a successively smaller postsynaptic EPSP. This mechanism is clearly homosynaptic in that EPSPs in the same motor neuron, that have been habituated to one stimulus input pathway, do not decline when the motor neuron is stimulated over the nonhabituation pathway. It is also evident that habituation is a presynaptic phenomenon in that postsynaptic responsiveness remains unaffected except when the sensory neurons used to habituate a response are stimulated. Although habituation resembles PTP in that it is both homosynaptic and presynaptic, it is fundamentally different in that it is due to a *decrease* in the probability of neurotransmitter release and not an increase as in PTP. Again, calcium ion concentration may play a mediating role. Kandel (1981) and others have proposed that habituation is the result of decreased presynaptic calcium ionic currents that in turn decrease the likelihood of exocytotic release of transmitter from vesicles. In effect, each successive habituation trial decreases the number of quanta of neurotransmitter released. What is amazing and as yet unexplained is how such a relatively few sensory inputs can totally inactivate a presynaptic sensory pathway for periods of days or weeks.

As with PTP and habituation, sensitization, or responses to otherwise neutral stimuli following recent presentation of a very strong or noxious stimulus, also occurs at presynaptic loci. Sensitization, however, increases the amount of neurotransmitter (or number of quanta) released at sensory synapses that have not been stimulated directly. It is therefore a heterosynaptic phenomenon. It has been suggested, but not proven, that collaterals of the sensitization pathway may contact other sensory neurons and regulate their neurotransmitter release (Castellucci and Kandel 1976). As with the other types of learning, calcium ions play a determining role in increasing the probability of neurotransmitter release.

Classical conditioning appears to share a common mechanism with sensitization, i.e., presynaptic and heterosynaptic facilitation of responses. It differs, however, in that the temporal demands of classical conditioning require that UCS precede CS by less than a second. Unfortunately, the mechanisms of classical and also instrumental conditioning are only beginning to be elucidated in contrast to the short-term learning paradigms. It is of interest to note that several examples of postsynaptic facilitation have been described in relation to classical conditioning (Brons and Woody 1980; Matsumura and Woody 1980).

One study of instrumental conditioning mechanisms that deserves note is that of Kennedy (1979). He has shown, in Rhesus monkeys trained to adapt arm movements to unfamiliar resistances, that efferent output from the red nucleus (which chiefly excites upper extremity flexors) goes to the inferior olivary nucleus and onward to Purkinje cells in the cerebellum. Such olivary-cerebellar activity is present only during learning of novel arm movements. Once the movement is learned to criteria, resistance input, via spinocerebellar pathways, automatically elicits the learned compensation for an unexpected load. This is a demonstration that a specific neural circuit exists to "teach" the cerebellum how to automatically regulate movements.

At last, the discussion of the six paradigms of learning and their neural patterns and mechanisms comes to a close. Without apology, the information presented in this chapter represents a simplification and condensation of information that is far more complex in its particulars than it would appear from this presentation. The next chapter will apply much of the "basic science" information to clinical situations encountered in therapy. The six paradigms of learning will be employed to construct a general set of rules concerning the sequencing and conduct of therapeutic activities. Each reader should now be in possession of a new or at least modified viewpoint concerning how behavioral adaptations occur and what neural mechanisms support these changes. With this fresh outlook, we now turn to the ultimate purpose of this book—to promote increased therapeutic competence by considering *therapy as learning*.

CHAPTER THREE

Learning and Therapy: Approaches to Intervention

T he idea that therapy is learning is not novel. The 1972 AOTA Conference in Los Angeles featured a group of presentations on the theme of "learning theories," that were subsequently published in the *American Journal of Occupational Therapy*. Hollis (1974) reviewed earlier studies concerning operant conditioning and the conduct of therapy, and observed that the use of such explicit learning theory did not restrict the options of therapists or prevent them from being truly eclectic with respect to their treatment approaches. Her point, which is still valid, is that therapy is in some, but not all, respects a process which requires learning. On the other hand, she implied clearly that the converse was not the case, i.e., learning is not therapy. Simply stated, therapy as learning is only one aspect of intervention. Explicit analyses and control of learning variables have little or no value if the principles and procedures used in treatment lack validity.

Ethridge (1968) and Peck (1968) in their commentaries on an article by Smith and Tempone (1968) were critical of the lack of explicit and informed use of learning principles by clinicians. Ethridge implied that an explicit statement of learning principles and methods ought to be part of the treatment planning for every client. Peck deplored therapists' lack of detailed and specific knowledge of learning principles. Implicit in their criticisms was that the therapeutic process was most often, if not always, also a learning process. Ethridge and Peck suggested that therapists should have formal training in theories and principles of learning.

Ayres (1970) concurred on the need to educate therapists concerning the learning process, and suggested that there were three principles related to therapy that were of special importance: "... learning takes place as a function of reward and reinforcement; one learns what he does; learning takes place because there is a purpose for its taking place." Ayres' suggestions concerning the application of learning principles to motoric training followed Trombly's (1966) report on the application of operant principles to orthotic training of quadriplegic patients. Shaperman (1979) described how a retrospective analysis of the learning patterns of children with above-elbow prostheses could be used to develop a more efficient and effective training protocol. Abildness (1982) reviews both classical and operant conditioning as related to biofeedback and offers some practical guidelines for treatment. Stein (1983) devotes an entire chapter to behavior modification principles and techniques. Such examples illustrate the concerns of therapists with issues of learning. They also suggest the applicability of learning concepts to a wide range of therapeutic approaches.

This book was written to provide therapists and others interested in (re)habilitation, with a systematic overview of learning. It describes different types of learning and tells something about the neural basis of each type. This chapter is the heart of this treatise. It begins by raising issues related to the role of the therapist in learning and then discusses philosophical and ethical issues. This is followed by a discussion of general principles of learning which apply to most, if not all, therapeutic situations. The remainder of the chapter deals with specific principles related to each paradigm of learning described in chapter 2. Throughout this chapter I have selected examples from those areas of practice with which I am most familiar: physical dysfunction, developmental disabilities, and sensory integrative dysfunction.

Every nervous system, from the simplest to the most complex, is genetically endowed with the ability to learn. Learning, or the ability to modify behavior as the result of experience, may be thought of as the alteration of an individual's response potentials as a function of *stimulus history*.

In theory, both *antecedent* stimuli, which elicit behavior, and *consequent* stimuli, or those that follow behavior and serve to act as reinforcers of emitted behaviors are capable of producing learning. The former includes PTP, PTD, habituation, sensitization, and classical conditioning; the latter refers to operant conditioning. Although behaviors of nonhuman animals have provided insights into human learning, this analysis will be restricted to human learning. Munsinger (1975) has identified four components of learning situations: drives, stimuli, responses, and reinforcers. Thus far we have described three basic drive states—*primary drives* related to tissue deficits; *secondary drives*, which are often cognitive and relate to socially defined "needs" such as achievement, attention, affiliation; and *competency drives* related to the "need" to explore, manipulate, and move effectively within one's environment. Above stimuli were categorized as antecedent or consequent, but can also be defined as environmentally produced (*external*), or produced within one's own body (*internal*). Responses may be classified in many ways, but the simplest distinction, that of either *reflexive* or *voluntary*, is most useful for present purposes. Finally, reinforcers are classed as *positive, negative,* or *punishment* as defined previously and are always *consequent* stimuli. Although much of what is presented may also be applied to psychiatric intervention, no attempt has been made to do so at this time.

The ultimate test of this material will be its utility. If it helps develop intervention strategies that increase the range of options, if it provides guidelines for improving effectiveness, if it gives a new basis for self-evaluation and assessment, and if it helps make decisions concerning the sequencing of activities and the nature, amount, and timing of feedback needed to facilitate learning, then it will be of value. Throughout this chapter those statements of principles or guidelines considered to have direct implications for the conduct of therapy are in italics. Readers who wish to explore these principles further should consult the references.

A simple description of learning components is useful as a point of departure. These will be discussed as they relate to short-term, intermediate, and long-term learning paradigms which follow later in this chapter.

Why define the components of learning situations? Even the most elementary therapeutic action or activity is highly complex. It is rarely, if ever, possible to describe fully all stimuli impinging on even a single alpha motor neuron, let alone an entire person. What is possible in the clinic is not a molar description of the minute events that are "learning" but a systematic consideration of the *types* of events and their *relative* (rather than absolute) importance as determinants of behavior. Likewise, drives, responses, and reinforcers cannot be appreciated in all particulars but only within conceptual categories that are useful to the therapist in making decisions concerning the activities, methods, and environmental conditions to be used in service of patient needs.

One important distinction is that of *overt* or *observable events* as distinct from *covert* or *unobservable events*. If attention is used to positively reinforce a hyperactive child's behavior of sitting quietly in a chair and working on a project, one might go over to the child, sit quietly nearby, and say "It's not easy to sit still for so long. I appreciate your working so hard on your project." The overt stimuli associated with this reinforcing event are the physical presence of paying attention. These include the visual stimuli of the child looking into one's eyes, seeing one smiling approvingly, and hearing words with a tone of voice that is low and even. Even the specific words, chosen carefully (*see* Ginott 1965), are overt, desirable stimuli. Yet there are important covert stimuli that also act as reinforcers. If the carefully selected words *elicit* positive affective response and a series of autonomic sensations that are pleasurable, e.g., bodily sensations associated with a positive affective state of happiness or pride, then both *overt* reinforcers and *covert* reinforcers (autonomic sensations) are congruent and one has successfully responded to an operant with a *set* of positive reinforcers. If, however, everything is done exactly as before and only the words are changed to say "You are such a good child. You can sit still almost as long as Max," the child's understanding of the meaning of one's attention may change drastically (Ginott 1965). All overt reinforcers may be positive, but the term "good child" may arouse anxiety (unpleasant autonomic sensations) at being evaluated and resentment (also unpleasant autonomic sensations) at being compared to another child. In this case *overt* stimuli are positively reinforcing but *covert* stimuli are negatively reinforcing and it is not likely that this intervention will contribute constructively to altering the child's behavior.

Using this same example, it should be noted that *attention* of the learner is also an important determinant of learning. If the child is preoccupied with bodily sensations or *internal* stimuli at the time *external* stimuli are presented as reinforcement, it is possible that the reinforcement will fail to be perceived and may not be interpreted as a consequence of previous behavior. In this case, both the novelty of the reinforcing stimuli (i.e., it cannot be a stimulus to which the child has "learned" not to respond—habituated) and the intensity of "stimuli," which will usually lead to arousal if increased sufficiently, may be critical in determining the child's *perception* of salient features of the environment.

Intrinsic neural mechanisms that are largely genetically determined prepare each person to learn from their environments and their responses to events. These mechanisms, which were discussed earlier, also dictate that learning will take place because of naturally occurring stimuli and responses. Certain responses are preprogrammed or "hard-wired" into our nervous systems. Stretch, postural, and protective reflexes all fall into this category. With such behaviors learning occurs *directly* in that there are many constant features of the environment (such as gravitational field) that operate to elicit behavior beyond any human control. The simpler an organism is, and the more reflexive its behavior, the greater is that animal's reliance on *direct learning experiences*. But another type of interaction between individual and environment exists, and is termed the *mediated learning experience* (*MLE*) and is described by Feuerstein (1979) as follows:

> Here the stimuli impinging on the organism are transformed before they enter into the system by another organism that interposes itself between the sources of stimuli and the organism receiving them. It is the interpos-

ing individual who mediates the world to the child by transforming the stimuli-selecting stimuli; scheduling them; framing and locating them in time and space; grouping certain stimuli or segregating others; providing certain stimuli with specific meanings as compared with others; providing opportunities for recurrent appearances; bringing together objects and events that are separate and discrete in terms of temporal and spatial dimensions; re-evoking events and reinforcing the appearance of some stimuli; rejecting or deferring the appearance of others; and through this, providing the organism with modalities of selecting, focusing, and grouping objects and events.

In humans, MLEs are an essential part of many developmental processes. All symbolic learning, be it verbal or abstract, that transmits social values or ideas must be mediated. Humans, much more than other animals, take an active role in selecting, defining, and presenting stimuli that will elicit and/or reinforce the kinds of behavior desired by the mediator, i.e., parent, teacher, social authority, even peers. With mediated processes, the primary learner will alter responses as a function of experiences, and the mediator may actively learn as well. Mediation is highly goal-directed. It seeks to establish patterns of behavior in the learner that provide not only for immediate modification of behavior but also establish general social rules of behavior. Direct exposure to stimuli is also important for human learning. Much motoric and perceptual learning depends on such experiences, which are often termed "trial and error" learning.

So far, the use of the term "teacher" has been avoided, and for good reason. Rogers (1969) said: "Teaching, in my estimation, is a vastly overrated function." I agree with this, but did not always feel this way. Teaching is the activity of a mediator. It is a process that at best evokes certain positive images of those "educators" we have each appreciated or admired in our past, and at worst evokes a wide range of negative feelings for those who, under the guise of teaching, have sought to control, manipulate, or restrict our learning. A therapist's most vital contribution is assisting people to learn those things they desire to learn; to help them learn how to learn best.

Treatment precautions, joint protection techniques, the parts of a prosthesis, and other therapeutic information which is esoteric to users may require therapists to be rather more directive. The most meaningful learning in therapy is that which is self-directed toward the goals of the learner. Therapists may augment or supplement experiences but there must always be a conscious effort to respect the self-defined goals and meanings of the learner. This does not mean that therapists must be passive or unobtrusive. If a patient wants to learn to do "wheelies" in order to jump curbs in a wheelchair, then the ideas, coaching, and reinforcements a therapist can provide will greatly simplify a process that could be dangerous and discouraging without that active involvement. On the other hand, if a therapist wants to *teach* a patient to do "wheelies" and the patient does not want to learn, they may both have unpleasant and unproductive experiences.

With adult patients, therapists often do conceptualize their role as that of a facilitator. (There are those, unfortunately, who have fixed treatments established for each patient, but such therapists who "set-up" their patients with meaningless or demeaning activities are in the minority.) Most therapists negotiate treatment options with patients. They attempt to learn the intrinsic needs (drives) of each person they seek to help and to define goals *with*, not *for*, their patients.

With children there may be a tendency to let the child's parents define learning goals to the *exclusion* of the child. One problem of working with children may be that clinicians act as *teachers* who impose therapeutic goals and structures on them, rather than as facilitators who assist children toward more competent play, self-expression, and social interactions. Although therapists often cannot sit down and discuss goals with children, they can observe their behaviors and make inferences concerning what the child is motivated or prepared to learn. They can also continually evaluate children's responses to their actions and assess whether or not their therapy is meaningful to the child. Certain assumptions are warranted on our part with children. If all primary drives are satisfied we may well assume that there will remain a need to explore, manipulate, and move within the child's environment. This is often a good starting point because we can provide novelty, fun and challenges as part of our intervention. If we start with secondary drives (often social) and do not know the child well, we run the risk of selecting reinforcers that are not meaningful. With exploratory play as a starting point we may better determine children's motivation by their choice of toys or activities.

Bandura (1969) reminds us that just as therapists facilitate learning through selective reinforcement of patient behaviors, so too do patients selectively reinforce our behaviors as therapists. Indeed, most learning situations are reciprocal rather than controlling. Therapists can be manipulated or enticed into being ineffective at times and should be alert to this. For example, the therapist working with a child who has sensory integrative dysfunction may discontinue balance and equilibrium activities if the child yells or cries each time the activity is presented. Such "punishment" may be interpreted by the therapist to mean the child does not like being there, or perhaps does not like the therapist. This leads the therapist to cease an activity and avoid undesirable experiences, i.e., to negatively reinforce themselves, and unfortunately tends to suppress the efforts of the therapist to help the child. On the other hand, a more viable interpretation might be that the child is not yet prepared or motivated for that activity and selection of less difficult or less threatening alternatives may allow the focus to remain on developing balance and equilibrium under conditions more favorable to learning.

Adults also influence therapists reciprocally. Patients who ignore us (i.e., nonreinforcement) may extinguish some of our actions designed to help them. If we simply term such persons "unmotivated" because they do not reward us for doing what we initially thought best, then we may tend to excuse them from therapy or pay less attention to them. Such an interpretation avoids the real issue. Unless we find out *why* our patient responded to us as described, we can't know how to help. It is rare, perhaps impossible, that a person is totally unmotivated. In most cases they are motivated toward ends that we have not considered or acknowledged. To say to a stroke victim, "I'm here to help you learn how to dress yourself" overlooks that the individual is demeaned (punished) by the implication, however true, that his or her functioning has reverted to that of a child. More significantly, it overlooks the patient's current goal which is to understand what has happened and to begin to reorganize self-definition and relationship to others. A more open approach on the therapist's part might be to say "I'm here to help. What can I do for you?"

Some therapists might say that this gives the patient the idea that the therapist has no definite role or cannot provide specific services— or it might give the impression that the therapist can do any and everything. Neither is the case. If patients ask for assistance that therapists can't render, they should be helped to find those who can help them. If the patient expresses conflicts over goals, help resolve those conflicts through listening and shaping responses that will define the patient's needs and priorities. If the patient expresses goals that are within one's expertise but that one is not motivated to perform, then evaluate your own feelings and beliefs and decide if you can assist this patient.

Therapy as learning is not mechanistic. It is not the unthinking, uncaring, or rigidly technical adherence to procedures. It is, in fact, not likely to be successful as a therapeutic viewpoint unless practiced in a humanistic context. The same ethical precepts and standards which apply to other therapeutic practices also apply to those which seek to facilitate learning. As Bandura (1969) has observed, an unethical practitioner might choose to employ behavior modification techniques to dominate or control a person's behavior, but an ethical practitioner would never do so. Therapists who subscribe to a philosophy that patients should be assisted toward independence, that intervention should be active rather than passive, negotiated rather than dictatorially applied, and that patients are to be treated with respect, dignity, and caring are not likely to abuse their role as facilitators of learning.

Relationships are essential to therapy. They are more than the sum of their parts, more than operant stimuli that reinforce behavior. With this in mind let us now consider general principles related to therapy as learning.

GENERAL LEARNING PRINCIPLES IN THERAPY

Not all behaviors can be explained in terms of learning, nor can all behavioral changes be ascribed to learning. Recall the definition of learning provided on the first page of the Introduction. Learning is the process whereby an individual modifies responsiveness to stimuli or acquires new patterns of behavior as a result of previous interactions with the environment, not including those changes due to growth, maturation, or aging, those caused by diseases or trauma, or those which reflect a change in levels of awareness or motivation. Bitterman (1975) has stated this as a general principle:

> Since performance in learning situations is determined by a variety of processes other than learning, differences in performance may be due to differences in processes other than learning.

Of what significance is this to the practice of therapy? First, many of our patients have had their nervous systems altered either *directly* or *indirectly* by disease or trauma. Direct alteration includes cerebral palsy, chronic pain conditions, spinal cord injury, Down's syndrome, cerebrovascular accidents, peripheral nerve injuries, and a multitude of other neurological insults. Indirect alteration may result from changes in behavior due to drugs taken to ameliorate primary symptoms and from biochemical and biophysical changes in the functioning of organ systems in the presence of disease (e.g., alteration in biomechanical integrity of muscles, bones, and soft tissues, all of which are responsive to mechanical stresses and strains as well as to neural influences).

Such direct and indirect effects on the nervous systems of our patients establish constraints both on what we can help them learn and how we can help. If neural pathways that mediate a given behavior are disrupted it is likely that some or all information needed to effect behaviors will be lost. At one extreme might be a client with cortical blindness resulting from a closed head injury. Although certain visual motor reflexes mediated by the lateral geniculate nuclei of thalamus and the superior colliculi may be intact, the client will be unable to respond to visual stimuli. Such stimuli therefore are a very poor choice for reinforcement because incoming information is absent. For this client facial expressions and proximity may be totally ineffective; whereas tone of voice, pitch, and volume and physical contact with the client may be the primary avenues of expressing positive reinforcement.

Therapists generally have recognized this principle as evidenced by evaluations including not only deficit assessments but also assessments of skills and strengths, sensations and movements available to elaborate behavior and be modified by learning. A thorough sensory exam, for example, is a sine qua non of evaluation for the child with sensory integrative dysfunction. Obviously integrative deficits can be ruled-in only if no primary sensory deficit is present. Even more important is to assess how these children respond to primary stimuli, to establish which are strong or preferred channels and which are weaker and less preferred. Such information is of great value in maximizing our effectiveness as facilitators of learning. Thus, although we may *train* a child using sensations that are less tolerated or appreciated, as in the treatment of tactile defensiveness, we would not use tactile stimuli as positive reinforcement! To the contrary, we would use visual and verbal reinforcers as rewards and avoid any heightened arousal or noxious stimulation that could occur from tactile stimuli which the child is not prepared to receive.

Genetically preprogrammed changes in individuals also may be powerful determinants of behavior independent of learning. Such changes fall into the categories of "growth, maturation, and aging." When dealing with the motor development of a child, therapists routinely evaluate postural and attitudinal reflexes to assess the "maturity" of the neuromotor apparatus. Independent of age, children can only learn movements voluntarily if they are supported by reflexive mechanisms that are automatic and dependent on the integration of subcortical and cortical structures which mediate specific responses. Although it may seem elementary, therapists must continually ask if the behaviors that they seek to shape and modify are within the capabilities of the individuals. It is not simply that attempting to learn responses which the organism is not prepared to perform will result in failure—what is more important is that the individual may perceive failure as nonreinforcement at best and as punishment at worst.

Though the examples thus far have focused on operant learning (which is by far the most common paradigm) this principle also applies to PTP, PTD, habituation, sensitization, and classical conditioning. This is especially true with reference to levels of awareness and motivation or drive states. For example, if a person is badly frightened, highly anxious, or otherwise in a state of high sympathetic arousal, attempts to initiate habituation training may be futile. This is because sympathetic arousal is intense and may in and of itself result in autonomic stimuli which sensitize the individual. Since sensitization is heterosynaptic it may affect pathways that would *otherwise* habituate fairly easily. For this reason habituation of responses to unpleasant stimuli, whether a procedure to "desensitize" unpleasant phantom limb sensations in an amputee or to "desensitize" phobic behaviors such as agoraphobia (fear of open places), must always begin with low arousal states and a relatively calm and reassured patient.

Learning theories generally do not account for another type of preparedness for learning, that is, the role of strategies, verbal and symbolic mediation, and superstitious associations. Munsinger (1975) has stated, ". . . *with older children and adults there is ample evidence that strategies and bizarre associations between stimuli and responses are adopted."* Many such associations are verbally mediated. When a child learns a novel task there may initially be no strategy involved. Yet as learning progresses children often self-evaluate their own performances verbally. That is to say, they "speak" to themselves using their thoughts and readily analyze actions. An adult facilitator may also contribute to this learning. Either the child or adult may at some point identify a strategy or performance principle that enhances the frequency of success. For example, when learning to shoot a basketball, a coach may suggest that "standing with your feet slightly apart, right leg a bit ahead of the left, and aiming for the rear of the basket where the rim attaches will improve accuracy." Without these guidelines, the number of trial and error repetitions required to learn this might be inordinate. It is also possible that low success rates early on would discourage (nonreinforce) further practice.

Adults in rehabilitation often have their own strategies for relearning skills they have learned previously. To force an adult with a stroke to "recapitulate ontogeny" because reflexes are at the level of an infant will both demean (punish) the client and ignore any existing repertoire of strategies to enhance learning. The existence of such cognitive structures (strategies) to support perceptual or motor learning is a major contribution that a patient can make toward participation in therapeutic planning and decision making. Therapists should seek suggestions from patients, listen to their strategies carefully, and encourage them to use these verbal aids to performance.

Self-evaluation occurs under most learning conditions. Rogers (1969) has stated the general principle that, "*Independence, creativity, and self-reliance are all facilitated when self-criticism and self-evaluation are basic and evaluation by others is of secondary importance.*" Therapists are aware of the dangers inherent in a patient becoming dependent on the therapist for feedback and evaluation concerning progress. When we sense that a patient is performing to please us, saying what they think we want to hear, doing what they think we want them to do, and manipulating us to maximize secondary drive reinforcement (approval, recognition, attention, friendship), we know that the patient is not being helped to become responsible and independent.

Less obvious is that a patient who is only reinforced when a therapist is present is relatively incapable of learning or practicing outside of formal therapy sessions. Because most patients spend only a few hours a week in formal therapy sessions, progress will be slowed considerably if the patient does not practice and self-evaluate (reinforce) what is learned in treatment. Not only does self-assessment increase the time that can be spent learning adaptive skills, it often is more accurate feedback than that of a therapist or facilitator. Why is this so? Reinforcement schedules administered by someone other than the learner can rarely take unobservable stimuli and behaviors into account. If I stayed up late at night and woke up with a hangover I might evaluate *any* effort at being productive as worthy of positive reinforcement. Someone who was unaware of my internal state might negatively evaluate me because, in their judgment, I did not perform as well as I had in the past. Likewise our patients often know when they are and are not putting forth effort, when they are or are not in pain, when mitigating factors affect performance. They are, in many instances, uniquely qualified to not only reinforce their own performance but also to augment or discount feedback from others.

When patients are overly dependent on the feedback of a therapist, positive reinforcement not only increases the frequency of the target behaviors we seek to encourage, but also reinforces dependency behaviors. This often means that a person may gain skills which could promote independence but fail to become independent once discharged because the patient was not motivated to be independent in the first place. This is an obvious conflict with our professional philosophy.

Related to the need for each learner to self-evaluate performance is the need for most therapeutic learning to actively involve the learner. Ayres (1970) states this principle as *"One learns what (s)he does."* One of the most important sources of feedback concerning learning is "reafference" or sensations produced by one's own movements. Moore (1980) has emphasized that active performance may be especially important because the human brain requires that "subcortical integration precedes cortical integration." Learning on the unconscious levels of the nervous system may be especially valuable early in training and/or rehabilitation in that it may permit the nervous system to better utilize genetically programmed mechanisms to their fullest potential before augmenting such learning with self-evaluation and/or cognitive strategies.

Prior experiences and learning on the part of patients can also have negative effects on new or therapeutic learning. Stated as a principle, *Prior learning which is erroneous, inaccurate, or inappropriate may interfere with new learning and make it more difficult to learn.* For example, how many clients have been taught that "exercise must hurt to be effective?" Beliefs that directly contradict scientific principles of human behavior, physiology, anatomy, biochemistry, etc., may fail to prepare patients for the skills they seek to learn. This is one reason why a careful history and interview of each patient is important. Not only should questions be asked concerning the nature, extent, and results of prior therapies, but also the patient should be asked to comment on what is known about the present condition and how it should or should not be treated. By encouraging patients to discuss their ideas and reactions to the total therapeutic process, it is often possible to identify and remediate any misconceptions that would interfere with learning. Holt (1981) notes that the present "information explosion" has distinct implications for medical practitioners in that information that is accurate is being revised so fast that many people fail to keep pace. So too, much of the information comes from "experts" whose credentials are often limited to personal experience, whose methods are questionable, and whose motives are clearly self-serving. In case there is any doubt that such problems exist I urge the reader to check diet and exercise books at the local bookstore and to watch the commercial and cable television programs devoted to these subjects.

Individuals who seek help for acquired conditions such as accident and disease-related deficits may experience special problems related to learning. Loss of physical, perceptual, and cognitive abilities is often emotionally overwhelming, especially initially. For many persons loss of function threatens their body image and their sense of "self." It is important to be aware of this when planning treatment and helping such victims learn to accept and adjust to a radically altered self-image. A useful principle is *Learning that alters a person's lifestyle or behavior may be resisted if it threatens the individual's concept of self.* Often a person will want to "get better" or "recover" or "improve" but may not be able to accept the changes in behavior needed to do so. For example, many spinal cord injured patients are threatened by attempts to improve wheelchair mobility and skills because they see such learning not as improvement but rather as a final stage in being transformed into a "cripple." Therapists need to be sensitive to this issue and be willing to let patients select and direct learning rather than imposing a fixed set of rehabilitation tasks.

Another danger inherent in trying to help others learn is that the facilitator may interpret the behaviors and perceptions of the client in light of the therapist's own biases. Moore (1980) remarks sadly that:

> Very quickly the patient learns what the experts desire to hear, see or feel. This, of course, reinforces and perpetuates established biases and erroneous concepts concerning the N.S.'s ability to reorganize and recover (to some unknown degree) over a prolonged period of time. Similarly this "tuned-out" atmosphere sets up a climate of sensory deprivation, not only for the expert but more so in regard to the patient and his/her nervous system's potentials.

A general principle to minimize such biases is, *To successfully facilitate learning in another, one must be aware of one's own personal beliefs and biases and set these aside so that the patient's own perceptions and viewpoints may be fully appreciated.* I don't advocate being without biases, only that they be suspended when one *listens* to the learner. It is the attitude of acceptance and tolerance of ambiguity, even confusion, that is most important. As therapists we may desire so strongly to "do something" to help others that we force all available data concerning that person into our own preconceived categories and interpretations. This reduces our own cognitive load to comfortable levels, but it may obscure or distort what the learner wants us to understand. I do not believe that any person can ever fully "understand" another person. Such intimate and complete knowledge of another is a goal that cannot be achieved. What we can do is "be understanding," behave in ways that communicate our desire to know and appreciate others, our willingness to listen openly, and our nonjudgmental acceptance of them as another person. This doesn't mean that we accept or are nonjudgmental concerning their actions. Just because I accept that someone could be angry enough with me to hurt me doesn't mean that I will let them.

When therapists use the same methods, the same evaluations, the same activities with persons having similar problems they communicate a lack of desire to appreciate the patient as a unique individual. Even worse, they narrow their own range of available responses and interventions to a menu of behaviors that may at best lead to limited success as a facilitator of learning.

Earlier I observed that self-evaluation may be of equal importance to the evaluations of others. I have also stressed the need for active participation of the learner in any effort to modify behavior. The next general principle at first appears to contradict my earlier statements but is not at all incompatible with any principle discussed thus far. The great weight of research evidence as reviewed by Singer and Pease (1978) and Yu (1980) suggests that with respect to perceptual-motor learning (or sensorimotor learning) that, *Guided learning, i.e., learning that is organized and managed by a coach, teacher, therapist, or facilitator, produces more rapid learning of skills than "discovery" or "trial and error" learning where the learner must develop skills entirely independently.* This principle provides a powerful justification for the role of therapist/facilitator. It does not suggest that the facilitator *control* the learner, nor that learning should not be active, self-initiated, and self-evaluated. It suggests that "two heads are better than one" in that the organization and management of learning can and should be entrusted to a person with special skills while the learner is left to focus on the task itself. Yu (1980) has reviewed both animal and human studies of recovery from central nervous system lesions and concludes that, ". . . functional recovery or improvement beyond the level of spontaneous recovery can be obtained through training."

Where two (or more) persons collaborate to select, direct, analyze, and interpret learning experiences there are excellent opportunities to eliminate personal bias, to detect and correct erroneous behaviors, and to faithfully and accurately reinforce responses according to the optimal schedule for the desired goal.

In addition to all requirements of learning discussed so far most complex skills also require considerable amounts of practice. Cross (1967) defines practice as, ". . . performance of any overt or covert act one or more times with a view to fixating or improving the spatial and temporal organization of the same or any other act." Practice is not merely repetition of behavior, but rather repetition with specific goals. For behavior that needs to be stable and relatively invariant the goal is to closely duplicate ideal performance and eliminate variations from trial to trial. For coordinated movements that require the alignment and synchronization of body movements with changing features of the environment, the goal is to match changes in performance with changes in the environment. Simple examples of relatively invariant behavior might be shooting a basket or tying shoe laces, whereas examples of variable performance demands would include playing ping-pong and handwriting. Freud (1940) observed that practice differed from mere repetition in that with practice each recurrence of an action provides the opportunity to view performance from a slightly different angle. This is important not only to critically detect, analyze, and correct errors but also because it leads to enhanced generalization of learning, which will be discussed later.

Using the Cross definition of practice, a general learning principle is that: *Perceptual and/or motor learning requires practice; specific practice schedules need to be prescribed to maximize efficient learning of skilled responses.*

Cross (1967) cautions that practice should not be confused with exercise. He states that exercise is ". . . repetitious performance of an already learned act with the purpose of modifying in some way one's physical characteristics (musculature, physical strength, or physique)." He suggests that to benefit from exercises they must be learned, i.e., practice is needed to stabilize and reproduce exercise movements. Beyond the early stages of exercise training, practice, as defined by Cross, is relatively unimportant.

Skill learning, however, requires true practice. Crossman (1959) and Kottke (1980) provide evidence that perceptual-motor skill development may require a minimum of thousands of practice repetitions to learn a new skill and two to three million practice repetitions to reach maximal performance skill. These studies did not focus on trained athletes, but on female production workers in a cigar factory and patients receiving physical rehabilitation, respectively. Kottke concluded that it took thousands of practice trials to learn the pattern of skilled movements or coordination of movements and millions of practice trials to maximize dexterity or speed of coordinated movements.

When Kottke wrote the late Sidney Licht, M.D., to share these data with him, Licht responded, "I believe you. However, do not publicize this information. The idea that the development of coordination requires millions of repetitions is so overwhelming that therapists will be too discouraged to try to develop coordination in their patients." (Quoted in Kottke 1980). When I first read this several years ago I was horrified and offended. I had been aware of the Crossman (1959) data for some time and I knew that thousands upon thousands of practice repetitions *might* be needed to re-establish skills, just as they were needed to establish them in the first place.

My immediate thought was that this was a gross insult to the intelligence and ingenuity of therapists. One of the reasons I have always used board games and recently switched to electronic and arcade-style computer video games is that they require many repetitions, often very simple, within a short period of time. The games are not inherently therapeutic, but if I observe my patient's performance closely I can provide feedback, strategic or coaching suggestions, and reinforcement beyond that inherent in the game. I suspect that many therapists know the practice requirements of skill development, but do all therapists understand them?

Not only must practice be provided to learn perceptual-motor skills, but it must also be structured appropriately. To effectively structure practice requires that the learning facilitator have knowledge of and skill at task/activity analysis. With each skill to be learned, three questions concerning the structure of an appropriate practice schedule for learning the task are raised. First, should the learner practice the entire task or should the task be broken into component parts to be learned separately at first and later chained into performance of the whole task? Second, how should the time intervals between practice trials be spaced to minimize problems such as fatigue or forgetting what was learned earlier? Finally, should the task be practiced in its natural serial order or should this be reversed? Let's examine each of these questions.

The first question is concerned with the distribution between whole-task and partial-task practice. With whole-task practice, a skill is repeated in its entirety from beginning to end, over and over until the learning goal is reached. Partial-task approaches to practice are more complex as described by Cross (1967):

> The part-task practice technique has been further divided into subcategories—generally three. In the pure-part method each part is separately learned to a criterion, after which all the parts are repeated as a sequential whole until the whole has been brought to the criterion already attained by

each of the separate parts. Under progressive-part practice, parts A and B are mastered separately and then combined. Next part C is learned separately and then practiced with A and B. Parts are progressively added in this way until the individual is practicing the entire task. Repetitive-part practice involves progressively adding to the practice task parts which have not had the benefit of prior practice. That is, after part A has been learned, part B is added without having been practiced previously. Part C is added only after the unit A plus B has been learned to a criterion.

What guidelines exist to determine the appropriate approach to a given task from among these options? A task analysis of certain activities suggests that they are unsuited to being practiced other than in their entirety. Balance and equilibrium skills for example, or ambulation skills where one would fall or have to be rescued by the therapist or other helper if practiced in parts are best suited to whole task approaches. Handwriting, however, is best practiced initially as partial tasks due to both the complexity and highly variable nature of this skill.

Whether one selects whole-task or a partial-task approach also has implications for reinforcement schedules which must be taken into account in deciding which practice structure is best for a given person learning a given skill. In whole-task practice most or all of the initial trials are not likely to be performed successfully. This means that there will be few opportunities for reinforcement in early task learning and many more toward the late stages of practice. For older children and adults who are able to delay gratification, or for tasks that are extremely novel, fun, and/or exciting (i.e., intrinsically rewarding to be allowed to practice the task), or for relearning a task that a person has developed strategies for learning rapidly, whole-task practice will generally be superior to partial-task practice.

One option for using whole-task approaches when the above conditions are not met and the task is not suited to partial task practice is to use an interval reinforcement schedule. This initially provides frequent reinforcement for *persisting* at the learning task and reinforcement intervals can be extended (or eliminated) as proficiency in the task improves and success increases.

The longer the time interval between practice trials, the more superior is whole-task practice. Likewise, the shorter the intervals between trials the more appropriate is partial-task practice. This raises the second concern of how to select optimal time periods between practice trials (Fig. 27). The range of alternatives can best be conceptualized as a continuum ranging from maximally *massed* practice, where each trial is immediately followed by the next without rest, to maximally *distributed* practice, wherein the time intervals between trials are so long that what is learned has been extinguished or forgotten by the time the next trial occurs. Obviously, each extreme

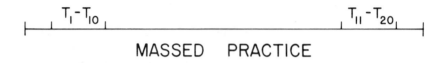

DISTRIBUTED   PRACTICE

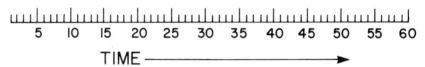

MASSED   PRACTICE

Figure 27.   A comparison of massed versus distributed practice (T = practice trial number).

of this range is to be avoided. The limitations inherent in massed practice schedules are fatigue and boredom. The limitations inherent in distributed practice are forgetting and the time, energies, and resources needed to set-up or return to the task.

Although no empirically determined guidelines for selecting from the range of massed versus distributed practice for specific tasks are available, such schedules should minimize fatigue, boredom, and the resources devoted to set-up of tasks and should maximize retention of learned skills over the total learning period. Whenever the time available for learning is limited or fixed, massed practice schedules have the advantage of producing greater learning because there is relatively less time devoted to rest and relatively greater time spent practicing.

Finally, the third question concerning the determination of an appropriate task sequence is appropriate whenever partial task approaches are employed. The options are either forward chaining of responses or reverse chaining (Fig. 28). With forward chaining, components of a task are learned in their natural order when performing the entire task. Those actions performed first are learned first and those performed last are practiced only when previous stages have been learned. With reverse chaining, the exact opposite sequence is employed.

For some activities reverse chaining is actually the natural or pre-

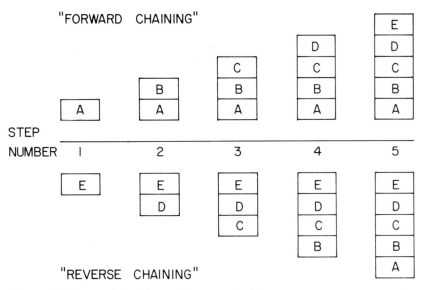

Figure 28.   Forward chaining and reverse chaining sequences are compared for a five-step task.

ferred method of learning. Bike riding is an example of this. Typically, children do not first learn to mount the pedal of a bike, swing their leg over, and then balance and pedal away. Such whole task practice is not as commonly employed as reverse chaining in which the activity is broken into two tasks: mounting and riding. Often the parent or instructor will help the child onto the bike, balance them, and then let the child practice the last step—riding off—first. Once the child learns to maintain balance and propel forward, mounting and gaining balance are practiced.

The selection of forward versus reverse chaining also has implications for reinforcement. When people are learning a task so as to gain or regain independence, they may negatively evaluate themselves whenever they find it necessary to depend on another person for assistance. Forward chaining always necessitates that the task either not be completed as part of practice until the final steps are added (as with partial task practice) or that, if the task is completed, someone else will have to assist. This means negative self-evaluation may occur at the end of every practice session. With reverse chaining there may be initial dependency but the person always finishes the task independently, and thus may evoke positive self-evaluation. Though actual rates of extrinsic reinforcement may be equal, the overall judgment of the patient in the forward chaining situation is "I can't finish it without help," whereas in the latter the judgment is more likely to be "I may need some help to get started, but I can do the rest myself." An excellent example of the relevance of this to clinical training would be a quadriplegic patient learning to eat independently. If therapy starts with learning to pick up a spoon using a tenodesis grasp and the patient is fed by someone else (not a pleasant or rewarding experience) it may take many weeks before the client really feels good about eating. Moreover, because grasp is more difficult to achieve than shoulder motions, the task is structured opposite the sequence of recovery of skilled movements. On the other hand, if the patient starts learning to eat with a universal cuff and mobile arm supports, then eating is self-controlled—relatively pleasurable and logically sequenced to use stronger, better controlled proximal musculature first. Reverse chaining in this example is the logical choice of most therapists for just these reasons.

In learning a perceptual-motor skill the patient needs to be aware that it may take thousands of repetitions to gain even a low level of skill. Rather than discouraging learners, it lets them know that they will have to practice repeatedly and consistently to reach their own goals. Someone who unrealistically expects to get better with one or two training sessions is quickly disillusioned and discouraged when no major gains in skill occur early in therapy. On the other hand, the patient who is realistic in outlook knows that initial gains will be small and that *persistence* and *repeated efforts* are accomplishments to be rewarded as much as skilled movement.

Another general principle deals with the relationship of events in the clinical environment to events in the natural environment of the learner. This raises the issue of generalization of learning, which is the degree to which learned behaviors can be elicited and/or reinforced under conditions not identical to those used in training. We may speak of either stimulus generalization or response generalization. Stimulus generalization implies that stimuli similar to those used in training will elicit learned responses (classical conditioning), reinforce emitted or voluntary responses (operant conditioning), or fail to elicit habituated responses. Response generalization implies that the same classical or operant stimuli or habituated stimuli may be effective with responses resembling those during training but more appropriate to the learner's environment. Figure 29 shows gradients or curves of stimulus generalization for two different classically conditioned responses—one shows a high degree of stimulus generalization, i.e., a wide range of stimuli not presented in training but resembling the conditional stimulus (CS) also elicit the conditional response (CR), and the other shows a low degree of stimulus generalization, i.e., even stimuli which are extremely close to the CS fail to evoke the CR most of the time. Similar generalization curves can be constructed to describe response generalization. A general principle of all therapeutic learning is that *Learning environments, practice sched-*

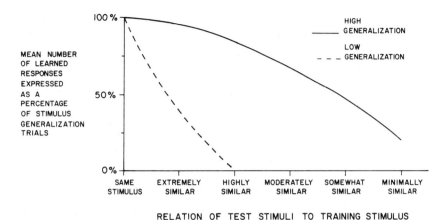

Figure 29. Gradients of stimulus generalization of conditional stimuli or training stimulus to other stimuli for a high generalization and low generalization task.

ules, reinforcement procedures, and learning activities must be selected and structured to maximize the generalization of learning from the training or clinical environment to the natural environment of the learner. How can this be achieved in therapy?

The point made by Freud cited earlier is most important. A critical element of effective practice is that it enables the learner to ''see'' the task from different angles. By varying the learner's responses, the nature of the reinforcement provided, and even eliciting stimuli provided by the facilitator or teacher, the learner comes to appreciate not only the requirements of skilled movement, but the dimensions of performance that are relevant and irrelevant. It may not matter if I chew gum while learning to shoot a basketball, but it certainly will matter if I am learning to play the tuba! Laboratories, where stimuli are rigidly controlled and responses defined operationally, may be appropriate to *studies* of learning but they rarely are appropriate for the learning of skills that are needed in a natural environment.

When we encourage a child with sensory-integrative dysfunction to throw a ball with both hands, we don't use the same ball at the same distance, to the same trainer, in the same room, using the same activity every time. We vary the ball, the task or game, and other stimuli and responses because our goal is to teach a general class of responses—bilateral throwing—not a splinter skill. A secondary and often covert goal of therapeutic learning is to help the learner discover *how* to learn—the process itself—so that if demands arise that the patient has not encountered in therapy it will be possible to analyze the situation and develop a suitable learning strategy and structure even without a facilitator's assistance.

Simulation, which Cooper (1979) defines as ". . . the creation of a situation that mimics processes or conditions that occur in real life," is an important learning technique in therapy. It provides opportunities to gradually shape learning by making the activities to be practiced more and more realistic as the learner gains skill and confidence. In the case of a disabled homemaker with acute rheumatoid arthritis, the therapist might suggest practicing joint-protection techniques and energy conservation during a simple task such as heating a can of soup. Later, the patient may be asked to plan and prepare an entire meal using adaptive equipment in the simulated "kitchen" of an activities of daily living (ADL) clinic. Finally, either on a trial visit home before hospital discharge or as an outpatient, the patient is asked to practice preparing meals at home. It is only by practicing a *range of adaptive responses* under a *range of stimulus conditions* that we can both assess and improve the generalization of learning.

Of course, to simulate the conditions of someone's home or workplace we must assess the salient features of those environments and closely replicate them in our clinical settings. To do so requires that we analyze the skill(s) to be learned, the person's abilities/disabilities, and the important stimuli and responses for the particular learning goals.

Another important method to maximize generalization of learning is postintervention follow-up. It is important to continue assisting patients with learning after they reach criterion levels of performance or goals that they have established. Inasmuch as forgetting, extinction, nonreinforcement, and many other factors can lead to some decline in skill it is wise to schedule a series of follow-up visits with each patient. For example, when I provide a hand splint I instruct the patient how to put it on and remove it, how to care for it, and when to wear it. I often ask to see the patient 2 weeks later to assess how the splint is being put on/removed, whether it has been cared for (or worn at all), and what wearing schedule is actually being followed. Any errors in component tasks can be corrected and the patient can be reinforced for being diligent. If a patient has not worn the splint I look for any possible punishment that it may provide or for competing behaviors which are being rewarded to a greater degree than wearing the splint is rewarded. I assume that if patients can not or do not learn what they say they want to learn there must either be conflicts that require resolution or other learning is interfering.

If I fail to follow-up on patients, I lose my major source of positive reinforcement—long-term improvements in the lives of those I help. I also lose the opportunities to correct my own errors or to modify the environment of the patient so that success will be possible. Often I find that further instruction is needed for situations that I did not anticipate the learner would encounter. I remember one paraplegic client with whom I did extensive simulation training concerning social and recreational skills, bowel and bladder programs, and mobility. We went so far as to visit nightclubs together so that he could practice his social skills, challenge his bladder with a few beers, learn to use public restrooms, and be able to maneuver his wheelchair in public. At our first outpatient visit about a month after discharge I asked him if he had been out at all. He replied only once and that it was a disaster. His favorite local hangout was a bar where patrons went up to the bartender, ordered drinks, and took them to a table. At first the bartender couldn't see him over the bar and when he did it was difficult to order because he had to practically shout he was so far away. Then he realized he didn't know how to get a full mug of beer to a table in a wheelchair, and he placed it between his legs splashing it onto his lap and embarrassed himself profoundly because it appeared that he had urinated (his greatest fear!). I had only taken him to my favorite bar where a cocktail waitress took our order at a table and served us our drinks!

It took about 10 min to practice pulling to enable him to stand at a "bar" (we had already used some of the required skills to practice pivot transfers), and a look through several catalogs found a wheelchair-mounted beverage holder. The next time I saw this patient he had once again become a regular at his favorite bar—and was also in technical school learning a trade. The point is that follow-up visits are an important part of assessment of the *outcomes* of learning and also a chance to further assist patients in learning to function independently. By gradually weaning patients from therapy rather than abruptly discharging them, the final outcomes may be more successful with respect to therapeutic learning.

The final general principle to be considered serves as a natural transition to the consideration of the six learning paradigms in relation to therapy. This principle is: *Shorter term learning paradigms should only be used when absolutely necessary to establish responses that can then be learned using a longer-term learning paradigm.*

Thus, if a patient can voluntarily emit a response which can be operantly reinforced, a therapist should not use PTP or PTD as a way of reflexively eliciting a response. Similarly, if responses can be extinguished through nonreinforcement, then habituation training is not warranted.

The logic of this principle is simple. When short-term learning approaches are used the patient must either frequently be retrained (which has financial, time and energy, and dependency implications) or later trained using a long-term approach. In short, we want the longest lasting results relative to the time spent learning. This leads to a hierarchical ordering of the six learning paradigms. Post-tetanic potentiation and PTD should only be used when behavior cannot be modified by intermediate or long-term paradigms. Habituation and sensitization should be used only when operant or classical conditioning techniques are not effective. And both operant and classical conditioning are favored over all other paradigms whenever feasible. With this in mind we now consider the six learning paradigms in relation to therapy.

SHORT-TERM LEARNING AND THERAPY

The short-term learning paradigms that are relevant to therapy are PTP and PTD. Basic features of each of these types of learning are discussed in chapter 2. Relationships between tetanic stimulation and behavioral changes in living organisms have received little attention compared to all other types of learning. Human studies of PTP and PTD are rare and have generally been directed toward evaluation of the effects of anesthesia rather than as studies of motor learning (Hutter 1952; Gissen and Katz 1969; Lee et al. 1977). What is presented here are possible, but not proven, relationships between facilitation/inhibition procedures and PTP/PTD.

One strong piece of evidence to suggest that certain of the so-called facilitation/inhibition techniques (see Farber 1982; Trombly 1983 for descriptions of these procedures) may represent examples of PTP and/or PTD is their remarkably similar time course. Just as with PTP and PTD certain facilitation/inhibition techniques lead to a transient change in behavior lasting from seconds up to minutes. The stimuli that elicit such changes are typically applied for 10-30 sec and only rarely for longer than 10-20 min. Like PTP and PTD, the responses affected are generally limited to those muscle groups whose myotomes correspond to the dermatomes via which the facilitation or inhibition stimuli enter the nervous system.

Another similarity with PTP/PTD of some of these techniques is that they display a phenomenon termed "rebound," in which a change in the desired direction of behavior lasting 2-20 min may be followed by a period of reversed effect or "rebound" in which clinically undesirable changes in the same behavior are present. Overshooting the pretraining baseline of behavior as the effects of PTP/PTD subside is commonly reported (Kandel 1976).

Figure 30 illustrates the phenomenon of rebound. Part A shows that a period of change in behavior in the desired direction will not simply return to baseline level 0 but will lead to a period of undesirable behavior. This undesirable phase of response to stimulation is the rebound phase. Part B illustrates the relationships of stimuli and responses during PTP wherein a brief period of tetanization leads to supranormal responses that gradually decline until they are actually

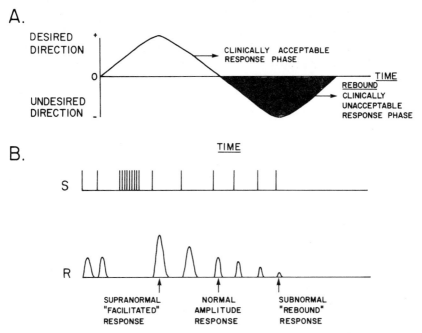

Figure 30. The phenomenon of rebound. *A*, shows the distinct phases of desirable and rebound responses; *B*, shows the relationship of stimuli and responses during PTP leading to an initial supranormal response and followed later by a subnormal "rebound" response.

subnormal. This subnormal response is the "rebound" response in PTP.

I have been careful to state that *certain* of the facilitation/inhibition techniques may represent PTP/PTD. Other facilitation/inhibition techniques represent either reflex activation, sensitization, or habituation. Reflex techniques are those in which the training stimuli lead to a single, short latency response that does not persist when the stimulus ceases. For example, the use of pathologic reflexes to elicit responses is advocated by Brunnstrom (1970) for flaccid hemiplegia. By giving resistance to motion on the relatively unaffected side of a stroke victim it is at times possible to evoke a mirrored (upper extremities) or reciprocal (lower extremities) movement of the more involved side. Resistance as advocated by Rood, Brunnstrom, Knott and Voss, and even the Bobaths ("placing and holding") as a sensory stimulation technique is also a reflexive procedure which utilizes stretch reflexes for either load compensation to maintain a movement or for enhancement of motor unit recruitment through muscle lengthening (Trombly 1983).

Quick stretch, a facilitation technique for the muscle which is stretched or an inhibition technique for the antagonist of the stretched muscle, seems to have both a reflex effect and a longer-lived sensitization effect that will be discussed later. Slow stroking of the posterior primary rami as described by Stockmeyer (1967) and other forms of repetitive, low intensity, non-noxious stimulation may in part represent the habituation of responses.

Vibration appears to have both a reflexive component, the tonic vibration reflex (Bishop 1974) and a component that may represent PTP/PTD. Although vibration is perceived via the pacchionian corpuscles as noted earlier, evidence suggests that the tonic vibration reflex is mediated via stretch of the muscle spindle. Frequency of IA primary afferent firing during vibration of a muscle belly or its tendon is quite close to vibratory frequency. Since optimal clinical benefits of vibration occur at 200 Hz (cycles per second) the requirements of tetanic stimulation are met. Farber (1982) gives an excellent review of the work of Bishop and others concerning the clinical indications, precautions, and methods for using vibration to facilitate target muscles and inhibit their antagonists. Unfortunately, she misleads readers in her interpretation of Bishop (1974, 1975) by saying that "vibration lasts only as long as it is applied." I quote Bishop (1974) directly, ". . . these positive effects of muscle vibration cease soon after vibration stops . . ." It appears that vibration may indeed represent PTP as well as a reflexive phenomenon. My own clinical experience with both quadriplegic and hemiplegic clients has shown that vibratory effects may provide enhancement of weak muscle contractions wherein such enhancement persists for several movement repetitions beyond stimulation. Effects such as vibration which potentiate or facilitate responses for even periods of 10-30 sec after stimulation are both clinically significant and within the temporal parameters of short-term learning paradigms.

Vibratory inputs also at 100–300 Hz lead to suppression of monosynaptic phasic reflexes. Gillies (1969) showed that the mechanism underlying such behavioral depression was presynaptic inhibition of IA afferents that synapse on spinal motor neurons. Again the stimulation pattern is tetanic and the mechanism is very much the same as postulated for PTD.

In 1979 I published results of a study of olfactory facilitation/inhibition stimulation using electrical activity of muscle activity as an indicator of altered muscle response to stimulation. Periods of 20 sec of relatively intense olfactory stimulation led to altered muscle responses in certain normal individuals that persisted more than 2 min beyond the period of stimulation. In the use of peppermint oil as a stimulus, similar 20-sec periods of stimulation produced depressed EMG responses persisting beyond the period of stimulation. The former data are suggestive of PTP and the latter of PTD as possible mechanisms mediating the short-term learning changes that were observed.

Studies of direct electrical stimulation of peripheral nerves (Beswick and Conroy 1965; Hayes and Clarke 1978) have reported that optimal longevity of PTP occurs with prolonged and relatively intense (850 Hz) stimulation. The minimal intensity showing augmented learned responses was 90 Hz. Although these studies were not conducted under clinical simulation conditions they support the finding that optimal vibratory frequencies of 200 to 300 Hz fall within an effective PTP range.

Whether such techniques are actually PTP/PTD is a question that cannot be answered at this time. The existence, however, of therapeutic practices which so closely correlate with these short-term learning paradigms suggest that it may be useful to tentatively regard them as such and explore the implications of this assumption for intervention. The goal of all therapy is to facilitate the learning or relearning of independent, competent, and meaningful behaviors.

To the extent that facilitation/inhibition techniques are purely reflexive, such as eliciting associated reactions in a hemiplegic patient, they lead to no behavior changes that outlast the eliciting stimuli. If no learning results then at best these techniques might be used to minimize the effects of disease on muscle and soft tissue, i.e., prevent contractures, slow down muscle atrophy. On the other hand, if reflex responses can be used to create new stimulus-stimulus associations, as with classical conditioning, then there may be beneficial results from using reflexes to develop associations that make it easier for a person to voluntarily elicit responses. As stated earlier, the general principle of using a transitory behavioral technique is that it be used only if responses gained by the technique are not available voluntarily, and will enable one to use longer term learning to more permanently improve performance. To use positive reinforcement following an elicited behavior is ineffective. First, the learner has not voluntarily emitted the response and, second, to receive a reward for something one had no control over is not positively evaluated by the learner. Instead, it may reinforce existing perceptions of dependency, hopelessness, and failure.

The great advantage of PTP/PTD over pure reflexes is that those methods that facilitate desired behavior (often muscle contractions) or inhibit undesired behavior (e.g., hypertonicity) for even brief periods beyond the application of the PTP/PTD stimuli *may permit one, two, or more voluntary responses that can appropriately be reinforced using operant techniques.* Even though the learner is clearly dependent on the therapist for the facilitation/inhibition to prepare for response, when such techniques lead to short-term learning (minutes) any voluntary responses which are thereafter enabled are clearly due to the person's own efforts.

The judicious use of these techniques early in therapy may have even greater value if they can be used to show someone with extreme weakness or paralysis that they do have *some* potential to control their muscles and move their limbs. In many cases, patients have tried over and over to move their limbs without success. Such nonreinforcement tends to extinguish further attempts to move. The patient may then give up trying. This in turn creates a self-fulfilling prophecy of hopelessness since the person often is less likely to care for the limb, especially if there is sensory loss. Subsequently such discouraged patients have a great risk of soft-tissue deformities and disuse atrophy of muscles. Should spontaneous recovery be occurring, albeit slowly, the results are even more tragic. The patient loses range of motion and strength, perhaps even allows weakened muscles to be overstretched by spastic antagonists, and is biomechanically unable to move even though the neural potential to do so has improved. This *masking of recovery* due to secondary biomechanical deficits has fooled even skilled neurologists into believing that the prognosis was far worse than is really the case. The techniques of Rood, Brunnstrom, the Bobaths, Knott, and Voss have all tended to minimize such erroneous notions by emphasizing the use of controlled sensory stimulation or facilitation/inhibition techniques for early mobilization of individuals with paralysis (Trombly 1983; Farber 1982).

Harris (1971) has provided an excellent summary of the relationship between reflexive and short-term learning techniques and other higher integrative processes:

> In certain cases, one may use facilitatory stimuli which produce their effects primarily through spinal cord circuits, but one is not only "treating the patient's spinal cord" in the process. Activity will also ascend to higher centers, e.g., reticular formation, cerebellum, and cerebral cortex, since every afferent fiber which makes spinal connections also sends ascending collateral branches to higher levels. At higher levels, the activity set up by the stimuli will be integrated with ongoing activity of other kinds. As motor responses to this kind of input are made by the patient, new patterns of sensorimotor organization should be built up in the CNS. As the patient monitors the muscle contractions and movements which result from the successful application of facilitation techniques, using visual and somatic (cutaneous, joint afferent, muscle afferent, tendon afferent, and so forth) modalities to pick up information from the moving limb, he will have an opportunity to strengthen or rebuild circuits responsible for feedback-controlled motor outflow. Or, as he regains the feel of normal muscle tone when he moves a limb in which spasticity has been broken up by successful application of inhibitory techniques, he will have an opportunity to reintegrate normal sensory inflow with his voluntary motor outflow.
>
> Of importance here is the effort of the patient to move actively during treatment if facilitation techniques are to be effective. If activity in descending motor pathways follows closely upon excitatory input of peripheral origin, both inputs converging upon common motoneurons,

the chances for successful discharge of motoneurons via these pathways should be increased.

Rood, Bobath, Brunnstrom, Knott, and Voss have always advocated that stimulation techniques be used only in conjunction with purposive and meaningful activities which permit the learner to subcortically or automatically *use* the improved responses. In effect, their rationale and methods are entirely congruent with learning principles even though they do not explicitly define a learning theory rationale for their procedures (Farber 1982; Trombly 1983).

Short-term learning has an important but very circumscribed role in therapeutic intervention. The very brief nature of such learning renders it unethical to use these techniques over and over to "teach" responses that will soon be forgotten or lost. Only in relation to longer term learning do these methods have a place in therapy. For this reason we now move on to consider habituation and sensitization.

INTERMEDIATE-TERM LEARNING AND THERAPY

Habituation has been described as the most ubiquitous of all behavioral modifications (Kandel 1979a, 1979b). Habituation serves to simplify the demands made on the nervous system by permitting organisms to learn to ignore stimuli that neither pose a threat nor reveal any new information about the environment. There is, moreover, widespread and general agreement that habituation is an important type of learning, both in and of itself and in relation to more complex forms of learning (Kupferman 1975).

Thompson and Spencer (1966) have listed nine principles concerning the characteristics of habituation. It is useful to discuss each of these in relation to implications for therapy:

> 1. *Given that a particular stimulus elicits a response, repeated applications of the same stimulus result in a decreased response (habituation). The decrease is usually a negative exponential function of the number of stimulus presentations.*

Habituation requires constancy of stimuli over a series of repetitions. The therapist must be able to control both the intensity and location of stimuli. Response amplitude tends to drop off more rapidly during early stimulation and less rapidly with later repetitions. Thus, although each successive stimulus leads to a decreased response, it may take more repetitions to extinguish the final manifestations of response than to reduce the behavior with early habituation trials.

The importance of this principle is illustrated in the treatment of childhood tactile defensiveness (TD). Low level, non-noxious stimuli under control of therapist or patient may be used to increase tolerance of tactile inputs (i.e., reduce aversive, defensive, or arousal behaviors). Brief periods of treatment lead to desirable changes in behavior, especially in the clinic. After several weeks of using habituation (stroking with light textures) there may be little appreciable improvement seen as behavior "improves." Negative behaviors may often be absent but will still occur even to low intensity touch especially if the child is in a state of heightened arousal (sensitized). The only way to extinguish TD behaviors more permanently is to continue habituation stimulation long after there *seem* to be no clinical gains in individual sessions. Unfortunately, therapists have failed to recognize habituation as one of the important neurobiologic mechanisms of remediation of this syndrome (Fisher and Dunn 1983).

> 2. *If the stimulus is withheld, the response tends to recover over time (spontaneous recovery).*

An important feature of habituation is that the longer a period of nonstimulation following habituation the greater the return to previous response levels. When treating tactile defensiveness in children or when using tactile stimulation to reduce adverse responses to unpleasant phantom limb sensations in amputees, it is most important that treatments be repeated frequently. It is advisable therefore to establish a schedule of distributed practice to minimize the "forgetting" of habituated learning.

It is common practice to measure how much habituation has occurred by measuring the amount of recovery that takes place following different time intervals (Petrinovich and Patterson 1979). Bishop and Kimmel (1969) compared retention of habituation to retention of longer term conditioning using nonreinforcement to extinguish responses. They found that the retention curves were similar for comparable numbers of learning trials, but that habituation was not retained nearly to the extent of conditioned learning.

Why not use operant treatments to remediate tactile dysfunction of the amputee or child with TD behavior? First, to extinguish behaviors via nonreinforcement requires that the behaviors be established by reinforcement. With defensive responses to touch, the situation is one of avoidance learning where the increases in excitability from unpleasant touch are reinforced positively by the avoidance of such noxious touch. Because nonreinforcement would necessitate preventing avoidance (presumably without negative reinforcement), the individual would undoubtedly become fearful of anticipated (although nonexistent) threats of noxious touch. These situations involve conditioned fears, so there is really little alternative other than desensitization (habituation) training.

3. *If repeated series of habituation training and spontaneous recovery are given, habituation becomes successively more rapid (this might be called potentiation of habituation).*

Not only do frequent training sessions mitigate against the loss of habituated learning, they also increase the ease with which responses can be extinguished during each successive training period. Habituation functions to eliminate undesirable behaviors and is rarely the final goal in therapy. Most often, as with the examples cited, habituation is used to alter behavior so that the person can better focus on *other* stimuli related to learning of skilled movements or perceptual or cognitive learning. Where most of early treatment time is used to habituate undesirable responses and little time for other training, repeated habituation easily abolishes responses in later sessions and allows larger and larger blocks of time for learning other primary adaptive skills.

4. *Other things being equal, the more rapid the frequency of stimulation, the more rapid and pronounced is habituation.*

This principle is closely related to the previous one in that longevity of habituation and effectiveness appear to be functions of the number of trials. One inhibition technique used with spasticity, that may be both reflexive and habituation, is the use of the hard cone to place pressure on the insertions of flexor tendons and maintain pressure on the volar aspect of the hand (Farber 1982). Because such devices are often worn continuously as splints, because they are low intensity, repetitive stimuli, and especially because there seems to be a decrease in spasticity as evidenced by increased range of motion of extensors *following* removal of the device, it may be that abnormal motor neuron activity is at least partially decreased by such prolonged stimulation.

5. *The weaker the stimulus, the more rapid and/or pronounced is habituation. Strong stimuli may yield no significant habituation.*

This principle suggests the importance of sequencing activities with respect to using habituation to extinguish adverse responses. Should initial stimulation be excessive, the child will be more likely to be sensitized and very unlikely to habituate. An excellent example incorporating this principle into sensory integrative therapy is given by Ayres (1972):

> Rapid spinning, especially without the requisite of an adaptive response, can be excitatory and also disorganizing because of its powerful effect and hence should be used only with careful attention to the response of the child. As with all other activities, the therapist is advised to try the process himself to experience the results of the stimulation. Slow, rhythmical, and

hence usually inhibitory vestibular stimulation can be achieved by letting a child lie or sit in the net hammock and swinging him passively back and forth or in an orbit, making about twenty-five or thirty revolutions a minute. Slow vestibular stimulation can also be given passively to a child lying prone on a large (thirty-six-inch diameter) therapy ball. The child lies passively on the ball while the therapist rolls him slowly back and forth. It is reasoned that the inhibition occurs in part through vestibular stimuli activating the cerebellum which, in turn, inhibits the brain stem, especially the reticular formation. It is also probable that brain stem centers governing vital functions such as respiration may be inhibited. A few undocumented instances of overinhibition through such procedures have been reported. This type of response illustrates the necessity for careful observation of a child's response to stimuli, especially of a vestibular type.

She continues:

Children with learning disorders vary greatly in their tolerance to vestibular stimulation. Some are afraid and their fear should be highly respected. The anxiety is interpreted to mean that they experience the power of the gravitational force as being overwhelming. Furthermore, they are realistic, for they cannot integrate the sensory input and respond to it in an adaptive manner. They are at the mercy of gravity, and gravity makes no allowance for handicapped children. It is appropriate for posturally insecure children to be fearful; the fear has survival value. To crawl into a barrel lying on its side is to surrender oneself to an unstable world that knocks one about at its will. A high place is dangerous if there is a strong probability of falling without the ability to land on one's feet.

Children with this type of reaction need a slow, safe non-threatening approach to the introduction and mastery of vestibular stimulation. Stimulation is introduced by the child's sitting securely in a net, hanging close to the floor and being encouraged to push the feet against the floor to begin swinging gently. The objective is to simultaneously increase the brain's capacity to integrate vestibular stimuli by developing the motor responses that aid integration and to gradually increase self-induced vestibular stimulation. As tolerance and the capacity to organize increase, the child can utilize the scooter board or the net hammock for more intense stimulation.

It is interesting to note that many of the empirically and theoretically derived approaches to sensory integrative dysfunction have little or no explicit learning theory rationale, yet they are often totally congruent and appropriate within the context of a learning viewpoint.

> 6. *The effects of habituation training may proceed beyond the zero or asymptotic response level.*

Clinicians who use repetitive stimulation to develop tolerance to tactile or vestibular stimuli, to decrease spasticity, or achieve any other therapeutic learning goal should always continue such stimulation beyond the point at which undesirable responses have disappeared.

This is because "excess" stimulation actually increases the longevity of habituation and allows for progressively longer periods of time in which desirable behaviors can be established via higher order conditioning.

> 7. *Habituation of response to a given stimulus exhibits stimulus generalization to other stimuli.*

Such generalization may be limited in that habituation is apparently homosynaptic plastic adaptation of the nervous system. What does happen is that different *events* that lead to similar patterns of action potentials in any given population of receptors are indistinguishable to the nervous system. Thus, there may be stimulus generalization in the treatment of tactile defensiveness which would allow a child who has learned to tolerate being stroked with silk to also tolerate being stroked with a cotton fabric. One would not, however, expect that stroking with silk would generalize to stroking with sandpaper! Such habituation could only be attempted following the serial habituation of adversive responses to less intense stimuli.

> 8. *Presentation of another (usually strong) stimulus results in recovery of the habituated response (dishabituation).*

A more direct way of stating this principle is that sensitization, which is a heterosynaptic phenomenon, reverses the effects of habituation. With respect to clinical implications, the passages just cited by Ayres suggest that intense vestibular stimulation may cause generalized arousal. It is therefore necessary to have control over the environment impinging upon the learner if one wishes to use habituation. Clinics that are next to the boiler room, directly in a major traffic pattern within an institution, or that have intercom systems used for paging and announcements may find at times that these make habituation more difficult to achieve.

> 9. *Upon repeated application of the dishabituatory stimulus, the amount of dishabituation produced habituates (this might be called habituation of dishabituation).*

The paradoxical implication of this is that, should one persist in attempting to habituate responses in an uncontrolled environment, one may be successful eventually if the sensitizing stimuli are repetitive and similar rather than random and dissimilar. Presumably the nervous system cannot be mobilized over and over again by a nondangerous, intense stimulus without learning (via habituation *and* associative conditioning) that the sensitizing stimulus does not predict harm.

Extensive evidence concerning habituation in humans exists. I have reviewed only a small portion of this literature which I feel has specific implications for therapy. Habituation occurs at all ages including

neonates (Stern 1979) although young children may appear resistant
to habituation partly because they have no prior stimulus history for
many types of sensation.

Even reflexes can habituate. Kandel (1979b) notes that Sherrington
had described habituation of the flexor withdrawal reflex in the first
decade of this century. Kupferman (1975) reviewed the literature on
human habituation of this same reflex in relation to both normal and
spinal cord injured persons. He suggests that both in health and at
least certain disease states reflexes may lose some of their obligatory
dominance over behavior, in part due to peripheral mechanisms—
i.e., habituation of spinal motor neurons and/or myoneural junctions.
This also suggests that therapists working with individuals with
delayed central nervous system development resulting in abnormal
persistence of primitive reflexes may be able to plan treatments to
minimize such reflexia. It has been said that there are distinct cervico-
cephalocaudal patterns in development (Moore 1980) and that higher
nervous centers must mature before they can inhibit reflexes mediated by lower centers (Fiorentino 1973). As a radical departure from
this, I suggest that the role of experience, especially habituation of
reflexes, has not been investigated as one mechanism contributing to
the organization and modification of the nervous system. I believe
that the success of the neurodevelopmental (NDT or Bobath) and
Rood approaches (Farber 1982) may be due in part to the repetitive
performance of tasks that may elicit reflexes repetitively, but always
in a context where they are constructive or purposive (operant learning). Likewise, even the Brunnstrom (1970) approach, which at times
uses pathologic reflexia simply to elicit tonus and contraction, may
contribute to the diminution of such reflexes via repetitive practice
that elicits these responses.

When one considers such possible contributions of habituation to
development of motor control or re-establishment of motor control, in
addition to the role of serial habituation in perceptual development
cited in chapter 2, it is reasonable to suggest that failure to consider
such learning may decrease one's understanding of perceptual-motor
skill development.

Jeffrey (1968) made three observations concerning the developmental role of habituation:

> First and foremost it was asserted that the control of selective learning and
> problem-solving behavior is primarily a matter of controlling attention.
> Second, a mechanism for the control of attention and the formation of
> schemata was postulated. It was proposed that a consequence of the ori-
> enting reflex (OR) is attending responses, which optimize the reception of
> stimuli. With repeated stimulation the OR habituates to a specific cue and
> the subject will shift his attention. As the result of such serial habituation,
> chains of attending responses (schemata) will be formed to cue sets in

which the habituation of the OR or two or more cues takes place in constant order. The third point was that if stimuli producing rapidly habituating OR's are paired with stimuli that produce OR's that habituate more slowly, the habituation of the OR to the first stimulus will be retarded.

A final piece of evidence concerning habituation comes from studies on lower animals. Caret et al. (cited in Kandel 1976) compared massed versus distributed practice in habituation. They found that both types of practice distribution permitted complete habituation of responses but that habituation obtained with massed training was not retained as long as habituation obtained using distributed practice schedules.

Before considering the role of sensitization in therapy I quote several passages by Ayres (1980) which describe a number of habituation procedures (even though Ayres does not overtly state this):

> Negative reactions are a clue that the child needs some extra tactile input that is acceptable. Sleeping between beach towels or in terry cloth pajamas may provide the tactile impulses that balance the activity within the nervous system. Or perhaps it will help to sleep with an extra pillow wrapped in a towel and lying beside him. Before the child goes to bed give him a light back rub. After the bath, give him extra drying with a towel. But watch his reaction closely; if he doesn't like the input, respect his wishes.

> If your child does lose his temper or self-control, punishment will only lower his self-concept even further. The child feels bad enough about losing control; punishment will make him also feel guilty and embarrassed. Instead of punishment, the child needs something that will help him regain his composure. A quiet place, such as his own room, away from the stress will help more than anything else. When the brain becomes disorganized, don't think punishment. Instead, think of controlling the sensory input from the environment to help organize that brain.

> First reduce the sensory overload, and second, provide sensations that are organizing. A furry toy, a favorite blanket, or a familiar pillow provide the type of sensations the child needs. Hugging or holding the child is even better for some children. Rocking in a rocking chair may help. For the younger child, a tepid bath may be soothing. Slow rubbing down the middle of the back increases the organization of the brain; do not rub up the back, for this moves the hairs on the skin opposite to their direction of growth and may produce defensive reactions. Outdoor activities will provide proprioceptive input that may calm the child's nervous system—especially if the weather is cool, since cool air helps to modulate the impulse flow from the skin and often reduces hyperactivity.

> Although therapy usually involves some self-direction on the part of the child, some sensory needs can be more efficiently met by the therapist directly applying sensory stimuli to the child. Brushing or rubbing the skin sends tactile impulses flowing to many parts of the brain. Tactile stimulation can have either a facilitatory or inhibitory effect depending upon which parts of the body are brushed or rubbed, and also depending upon

whether the stimulation is light or deep. The effects of touch are far more powerful than they appear to be. For this reason, untrained persons are advised not to brush the child's skin unless they are under the strict supervision of a sensory integration therapist.

Deep pressure sensations often help to organize a tactilely defensive, hyperactive, or distractible child. We often provide deep pressure sensations by putting the child between two mats to make a "hamburger." The therapist then presses down on top of the child, pretending to put ketchup, mustard, relish, and all manner of condiments on the "hamburger." Children often come out of this "hamburger" calmer and better organized than before. During other activities, the therapist may press the bones in a joint together or sometimes pull them to stretch the joint, thereby stimulating the sensory receptors in the joints.

Why are such extensive citations of treatment methods needed? If sensory-integrative, Rood, NDT, Brunnstrom, and PNF approaches already make such excellent use of habituation, why does it matter whether anyone has previously considered these to be habituation?

I believe there are several specific implications of *explicitly* identifying these methods as habituation. First, when one terms these "habituation" there is an implicit recognition that stimuli must be low-level, repetitive, and non-noxious. Since sensitization can occur it is *critically* important that the therapist or other facilitator (parent, teacher, etc.) be very *consistent* in providing sensory inputs. Any strong or sudden stimuli, such as yelling at a child with tactile defensiveness, may reverse previous therapeutic gains.

Second, the need to frequently and intensively repeat these treatments has not been stressed sufficiently. Especially noteworthy is the lack of instruction to continue these procedures long after the aberrant responses have ceased. Third, once one considers these techniques as habituation, one can develop a strategy to progress from the lowest intensity (amplitude) and least threatening stimuli to the more intense and provocative stimuli, i.e., serial habituation. Finally, inasmuch as habituation is homosynaptic, a variety of stimuli and environments should be used for training because generalization (transfer of learning) is quite limited with habituation.

I believe from my own observations, and recommend for further study, that treatments that *overtly* incorporate habituation principles rather than *incidentally or covertly* employ habituation lead to more rapid and effective adaptive learning.

Like habituation, sensitization can last for periods ranging from hours to weeks. As such it also is an important form of intermediate-term learning (Kandel 1979a, 1979b). Sensitization is a heterosynaptic phenomenon whereby a noxious or novel stimulus leads to increased responsiveness to a wide variety of other stimuli. Being heterosynaptic, it is neuronally more complex than habituation which tends homosynaptically to be restricted only to the stimulated pathways. Unlike habituation, sensitization is clinically simple. The stronger, more novel, and more odious the stimulation, the greater its effectiveness.

It appears that the most salient feature of sensitization is the widespread *arousal* that it induces. This is in direct contrast to habituation that functions to increase *attentiveness* and focus on relevant (nonhabituated) stimuli. Of what value is this in therapy?

My first example is from clinical experiences working with learning disabled and "minimal cerebral dysfunction" children. I was treating two slightly overweight, physically undeveloped, and quite fearful young 7- or 8-year-old boys. Both had been evaluated using the Southern California Sensory Integration Tests and found to have deficits of postural and bilateral integration (Ayres 1972) which today might be termed postural-ocular and/or praxic deficits (Ayres 1976). Both boys were extremely bright and verbal and tended to intellectualize and rationalize their fears concerning their bodies and movement. I found most treatment sessions to be a challenge in that they were quite sensitive to failure and afraid to take risks. I was therefore quite patient and proceeded cautiously for months to gain their confidence and to encourage and reinforce risk-taking and exploratory gross motor behavior.

One thing that annoyed me, however, was that neither child could climb stairs reciprocally. Since our "perceptual-motor room" was up a flight of stairs from our main clinic where the boys were brought for therapy, each session included a time-consuming (and for them frightening) ascent and descent accompanied by holding on to the bannister with both hands.

After months of sensory integrative therapy both boys began to make remarkable progress—during treatment and outside of treatment. Then one of the boys reported he could now ride a two-wheeled bike. What surprised me was how quickly this generalized to other areas, including stair climbing. The other child bothered me. I didn't want to think *I* had failed. In the therapy sessions both boys did well and showed marked improvements.

One day the time came to go up the stairs and the first child went up rapidly and reciprocally. My other small friend was still hugging the bannister on stair two by the time his companion had gained the summit. For some reason I still don't understand, I lost control of my temper and screamed (not spoke loudly—really screamed) at my laggard, and visibly upset him. I pulled him down to the middle of the bottom stair and in a near rage (by now all self-control was gone) *demanded* he ascend the stairs without the railing and reciprocally.

Looking back, I am surprised that I responded as I did. My young client did not intellectualize—he did not tell me I hurt his feelings or I was being mean (I would have agreed with him had he done so!). I presented a threat more potent than falling—I was *angry*! So without hesitation and with tears in his eyes he climbed the stairs reciprocally without holding the railing. Then he turned around at the top, smiled tearfully, and climbed down reciprocally! Thrilled with himself he ran down the hall, got his mother, brought her to the stairs, and, to her great surprise, went up and down perfectly.

I had *sensitized* responses which had been within his skill repertoire but never chained together successfully before that time. I was *credited* with getting my young patient to climb the stairs and was treated as though I had performed a miracle.

I have since learned that such sensitization was probably not luck. I must have been frustrated with the stairs because I strongly suspected he had the skills to climb them appropriately. With other clients I have also "gone with my feelings" and "exploded" (not a pretty sight), raised my voice, and mobilized latent responses.

Less dramatic as an example of sensitization is quick stretch, a facilitation technique of Rood and others (reported in Trombly 1983; Farber 1982). By shortening a muscle and then rapidly and moderately forcefully elongating it maximally, ideally just short of the painful range, subsequent responses of the muscle, especially voluntary, tend to be enhanced. Although stretch reflexes undoubtedly play a role in this augmentation they are insufficient to explain the endurance of beneficial effect beyond the initial period of stimulation.

Voice modulation, especially a sudden and unexpected raising of the voice, is a method of coping with progressive habituation of attention. The telling of jokes and use of humor have a similar arousal effect. Because such unexpected stimuli occur in situations where they are not predicted, they sensitize (arouse) responses and dishabituate orienting responses that have been habituated. To maintain high arousal and alertness during exams I employ exercise, such as jumping jacks, followed by jokes. This is well received by students as a relief from the tediousness of writing responses to questions.

With comatose, stuporous, and traumatic head-injured clients I have used sensitization procedures to *mobilize* responses when lethargy prevailed otherwise. Habituation and sensitization are complementary processes in that they strike a balance between focused concentration and generalized awareness. Both are nonassociative learning and both can last weeks, even months in some cases. Unfortunately neither alone is a basis for independent learning due to their impermanence. Only when followed by or used in conjunction with associative paradigms do these intermediate-term learning methods contribute effectively to therapeutic learning.

Long-term Learning and Therapy

Classical or Pavlovian conditioning has most often been used thera-peutically as a means of regulating autonomic nervous system func-tions. Abildness (1982) and Gatchel and Price (1979) have described special applications of biofeedback training which use combinations of classical and operant techniques to shape behavior for such prob-lems as headache, hypertension, cardiac arrhythmias, anxiety, and constipation.

Bandura (1969) has remarked that:

> Many problems for which people seek relief involve distressing autonomic overactivity reflected in a variety of somatic complaints of a functional nature, including chronic "tension" and anxiety reactions, gastrointestinal disorders, and respiratory and cardiovascular disturbances. Conditioned emotionality is also generally implicated, particularly during the acquisi-tion phase, in obsessive-compulsive reactions, behavioral inhibitions, and phobic and other avoidance behaviors. Depressant drugs may provide temporary relief from intense autonomic responses, but in cases where they are under stimulus control, social-learning procedures that are capa-ble of neutralizing the emotion-arousing properties of stimulus events offer the most direct and effective treatment.
>
> Autonomic responses can be most readily brought under the control of environmental stimuli through classical conditioning operations. If a for-merly ineffective or conditioned stimulus is closely associated with an unconditioned stimulus capable of eliciting a given physiological response, the former stimulus alone gradually acquires the power to evoke the physiological response or its equivalent. Although some types of auto-nomic responses are more difficult to condition than others, almost every form of somatic reaction that an organism is capable of making, including respiratory and heart-rate changes, increases in muscular tension, gastro-intestinal secretions, vasomotor reactions, and other indices of emotional responsiveness, has been classically conditioned to innocuous stimuli.

What techniques performed by therapists incorporate classical con-ditioning? With respect to motor control learning, the best examples come from the treatment of oromotor dysfunction in brain-damaged children and adults. Farber (1982) described a technique for the treat-ment of tongue thrust. Such a condition makes it difficult to eat because food is forced out the mouth rather than actively incorpo-rated by the tongue. One treatment technique is to grasp the tongue between moist gauze pads (a tactile CS) and quickly pulling the tongue into protrusion (a UCS) which then elicits a retrusion response (CR). The timing of this, wherein the quick stretch follows the grasping by perhaps 0.5 to 1.5 sec, is ideal for conditioning. Is this classical conditioning? My observations suggest that the repetitive application of this and other oromotor stimulation does lead to the CS-tactile stimulation—from spoon or food itself eliciting the CR.

Bowel and bladder training for spinal cord injured patients may use the association of the morning meal and sitting on the commode (CS) along with a suppository (UCS) to develop a pattern of defecation following breakfast that does not rely on suppositories. Note that the bolus formed 15 to 20 min after a meal also gives rise to afferent signals (UCS) that initiate the gastrocolic reflex which also assists defecation. Rovetto (1979) has provided ample evidence that this approach works in the treatment of chronic constipation in which coffee and the morning newspaper served as CS. More importantly a 1-year follow-up revealed that seven of eight patients so treated remained asymptomatic after several weeks of training.

A number of biofeedback techniques using imagery or autogenic training appear to associate the CS of images or words with stimuli such as regular deep breathing and alternate muscle contraction and relaxation that elicit a powerful parasympathetic reflex—the relaxation response.

These examples of classically conditioned responses involving somatic musculature are probably not the most powerful use of classical conditioning in therapy. I suggest that affective classical conditioning is more widespread than somatic conditioning. When patients work or play at tasks that are especially meaningful or pleasurable, it is likely that they learn responses to the stimuli of the tools and materials of these tasks (CS) which precede pleasurable autonomic sensations (UCS) which, in turn, give rise to motoric responses CRs (muscle relaxation, peripheral vasodilation). It is most probable that the UCS, i.e., pleasurable feelings, arise not from the activity but from the verbally mediated symbolic states wherein the mind says to itself "I like this, I always wanted to do this, I have fun doing this, I am excited to be able to do this." This is why one client often *loves* an activity another one *hates*. For each person it is their conscious assessment and evaluation of activities which determine the meaning, and hence the nature, of the UCS associated with these activities. The use of activity that *elicits* strong and positive visceral responses is an essential feature of all therapy and one that has led us to achieve positive results despite continued failure of neuroscientists to investigate the neurobehavioral foundations of meaningful activity.

Evans (1980) has reported on the classical conditioning of movements in neonates. The UCS of being picked up which via vestibular, tactile, and olfactory pathways can lead to a CR of decreased excitability and suppression of crying, when paired with the mother's voice can lead to the voice alone eliciting these soothing responses. Humans are genetically prepared to benefit from the natural associations of stimuli that exist in the world. Therapists can and should take advantage of such conditions when working with infants at risk for developmental problems. The use of limited and structured stimulation may greatly enhance an infant's ability to develop self-regulatory mechanisms.

To conclude the consideration of classical conditioning in therapy, we should remember that there is little *neural* evidence to suggest that the mechanisms of classical conditioning differ from the mechanisms of operant learning. For some learning theorists this has already been extended to include a blurring of distinctions with respect to behavioral differences between classical and operant conditioning. Hearst has commented:

> . . . "pure" examples of operant or classical conditioning are practically impossible to arrange. Whether the procedure is labeled "classical" or "operant," responses occurring in the presence of some stimulus are followed by a reinforcer. A variety of responses will be conditioned on either procedure and may interact with, interfere with, or facilitate each other. They constitute a whole pattern of behavior, and it seems misleading to call any one of them the conditioned "response." As we analyze the classical-instrumental distinction, the reader ought to keep in mind the above complications and interactions.

It must be recognized that most behaviors which therapists seek to modify are complex arrays of behavior made up of many stimuli and responses. Because classical conditioning requires that the therapist identify UCS, UCR, CS, and CR it is often more accurate to utilize an operant paradigm that simply requires that one be able to identify when a behavior has occurred and to what degree.

Of all the learning paradigms, it is operant conditioning that has been explored most in relation to therapy. Trombly (1966) has described operant training of orthotic control for quadriplegics. Solomonow and associates (1979) have reported that two-point tactile discrimination thresholds can be reduced using operant conditioning, with the end result that interelectrode distances used on augmented or prosthetic sensory displays for the blind can be decreased. This means patients can be taught finer discriminations for use with assistive devices that are electronically controlled. Shaperman (1979) has described the use of purposeful activity that would produce instrumental results in the early prosthetics training of child amputees. Murphy and Doughty (1977) report that contingent vibratory stimulation can be used with profoundly retarded students to improve control of arm movements. Burnside and associates (1982) have reported that a comparative study of biofeedback versus simple exercise therapy shows that although equal levels of skill can be trained with either technique, biofeedback training is highly resistant to extinction whereas simple exercise therapy is not. Fiorentini and Berardi (1980) have demonstrated that practice at perceptual discrimination tasks which are rewarded lead to improvement in perceptual task skills. Lucca and Recchiuti (1983) have reported data showing that isometric strength training is more effective when biofeedback is used to increase performance feedback than when it is not used. Harris and associates (1974) have remediated postural deficits with cerebral palsied children by giving them automatic reinforcement for using electronic signals to establish the location of their head and limbs in space. Hunt and associates (1979) have reported on the role of associative learning in habit formation and retention and suggest clinical methods of extinguishing undesirable behaviors. Even this brief sample of the literature related to operant conditioning and therapy demonstrates the expanding awareness of its role in clinical intervention.

Many of the operant techniques are considered to be behavior modification. Norman explains:

> Behavior modification is an approach for changing behavior based on a preliminary study of the individual. Behavior change is attempted once the individual's learning characteristics and the identification of the optimal learning conditions for the learner have been analyzed. The ability to analyze systematically and to develop behavior-environment relationships also brings a responsibility to the user to understand and master the principles and procedures of behavior modification.

A number of the basic principles of operant learning were discussed in chapter 2, and are expanded here. Operant learning is based on a principle that individual differences in learners determine both their motivations and which reinforcers will be effective. Although reinforcement principles are the same for all learners with respect to schedules, it is always necessary for the therapist to study carefully the individual client to determine potential positive and negative reinforcers.

Bandura (1969) has observed that the success of many reinforcement schedules can be enhanced whenever therapists share a knowledge of the process with clients:

> In most real life circumstances the cues which designate probable consequences usually appear as part of a bewildering variety of irrelevant events. One must, therefore, abstract the critical feature common to a variety of situations. Behavior can be brought under the control of abstract stimulus properties if responses to situations containing the critical element are reinforced, whereas responses to all other stimulus patterns lacking the essential element go unreinforced. It should be noted here that the controlling function of various social and environmental stimuli is usually established simply by informing people about the conditions of reinforcement that are operative in different situations, rather than by leaving them to discover it for themselves through a tedious process of selective rein-

forcement. However, the existence of differential consequences is essential to maintain stimulus control produced through instructional means.

When behavioral contingencies cause certain behaviors to lead to predictable consequences, the learner's knowledge of this will lead to a more controlled response.

I have mentioned that self-evaluation is of greater importance to a learner than the evaluation of a therapist. But I have also said that mediated learning or guided learning is more effective than "trial and error" approaches. Let me explain this apparent contradiction. Self-evaluations of specific tasks generally involve a determination after each task repetition of whether or not the task was performed successfully. Such a conscious evaluation of performance after-the-fact is termed knowledge of results (KR) feedback. Lucca and Recchiuti (1983) argue that biofeedback becomes a very special kind of KR in that it allows the learner to assess results not only at the end of practice but during practice as well. Reeve and Magill (1981) have shown that too much information in motor tasks may confuse the learner. They found that early in learning information about the direction of motoric errors was helpful to subjects as a form of KR, but that magnitude or distance of the errors was not useful KR information. Wallace and Hagler (1979) wanted to distinguish between final KR and intermediate KR (assessment of success during an activity rather than at the end). They continued to refer to final assessments as KR but have called intermediate assessment results KP or knowledge of performance. They compared the relative effectiveness of no feedback, KR, and KR + KP on the learning and retention of a closed motor skill (shooting baskets). They found that KR + KP was superior for both rate of learning and retention of learning over simple KR. Knowledge of performance involves a mediator of learning or facilitator since an individual often cannot stop an activity to assess how it is being performed. Knowledge of performance alone is insufficient information to direct learning without KR. Knowledge of results is thus superior to KP, i.e., self-assessment is superior to assessment by others. But KR + KP leads to maximal learning and retention and this is the situation that prevails in therapy, i.e, guided learning is superior to trial-and-error learning.

In conclusion, it is the role of the therapist to provide KP feedback to clients, to teach clients the response contingencies in operant conditioning, and to allow clients to perform their *own* assessment of KR. Regardless of the type of learning, the therapist must analyze and prescribe a *structure* of intervention as well as methods or activities. This brings me to the final section in this chapter—a consideration of how to effectively use the information I have presented to actually plan and structure intervention

TREATMENT PLANNING MODEL FORMAT

PROBLEM	GOAL	PRINCIPLES	METHODS/ACTIVITIES	LEARNING APPROACH

ABBREVIATIONS: *Problem*   *Learning Approach*
                 S = subjective   PTP = Post-tetanic Potentiation   FC = Forward Chaining
                 O = objective   PTD = Post-tetanic Depression   RC = Reverse Chaining
                                     H = Habituation   CR = Continuous Reinforcement
                                     S = Sensitization   FI = Fixed Interval
                                     CC = Classical Conditioning   FR = Fixed Ratio
                                     IC = Instrumental   VI = Variable Interval
                                          Conditioning   VR = Variable Ratio
                                     MP = Massed Practice
                                     DP = Distributed Practice
                                     PT = Partial Task
                                     WT = Whole Task

Figure 31.   Treatment planning format designed to incorporate learning variables into the design and structure of therapy.

Learning and the Treatment Planning Process

As I have advocated throughout this monograph, Therapy as Learning is a viewpoint or perspective on clinical intervention. Its purpose is to permit therapists to become more successful as facilitators of therapeutic learning by suggesting how and why certain sequences of treatment activities should be employed. It should also help therapists structure treatments so as to maximize long-term retention of learning. A final goal is to assist therapists in designing treatments that have a high degree of stimulus and response generalization built into the therapeutic process.

Since 1980 I have used a treatment planning format with occupational therapy students that requires them to explicitly structure the learning process as well as plan traditional intervention. Figure 31 shows the form that I ask students to use in preparing treatment plans and that I use with my own patients.

Note that under "Learning Approach" the six paradigms of learning are listed in order of increasing longevity of results. This is to remind the therapist that the selection of any paradigm, other than classical or operant conditioning, requires that the briefer term results be used to facilitate higher order planning. Next, the decision options regarding massed versus distributed practice and partial task versus whole task practice are made, and if partial task practice is selected, the decision whether to use forward or reverse chaining must be made. Finally, reinforcement schedules need to be designed whenever instrumental (operant) learning approaches are used.

While the development of a treatment plan which provides a structured learning approach does not ensure that the therapist will implement learning practices appropriately, it does establish a new set of standards for evaluating treatment effectiveness. These standards, unlike the more traditional aspects of the treatment plan, evaluate the activities of the *therapist* in conducting treatment in accord with learning theory rather than evaluating the client's responses to therapy. As such, it also acknowledges expressly the importance of self-evaluation to the role of the therapist as well as to the role of the learner.

The Validation and Discovery of Learning Approaches to Therapy

Therapists working to (re)habilitate children suffering from sensory integrative dysfunction, cerebral palsy, and Down's syndrome provide activities designed to facilitate developmentally appropriate sensorimotor responses. Likewise, those who work with brain-damaged or otherwise neurologically impaired adults also direct their efforts toward facilitating appropriate adaptive responses. It is the ultimate aim of all of these efforts to increase independent, goal-directed activity and to discourage dependency and disability behaviors.

Just as patients must learn the skills they need to master the tasks of everyday life, so too must therapists *learn* how to assist patients toward such goals. Although an extensive research literature concerned with learning principles and practices exists, there is a relative scarcity of literature addressed to therapeutic applications of learning concepts. Just as there is a need to document the effectiveness of our treatments, there is also a need to evaluate the principles and procedures used to deliver these treatments. The final chapter of this book is a brief statement of the needs for systematic investigations concerning therapy as learning.

Before therapists can claim to be competent to facilitate purposive movement responses they must demonstrate an expertise in motor and perceptual aspects of learning. Anatomic and physiologic studies of therapeutics (i.e., basic science research) is all too often retrospective and based on lesion studies that may not resemble clinical pathology. Prospective studies utilizing appropriate behavioral and physiologic measures are needed urgently.

Principles identified via the study of simple nervous systems may enable the identification of rules for therapeutic intervention with human clients. It is significant that the electrophysiologic properties of simple nervous systems, such as those of invertebrates, are nearly identical to those of higher organisms. We need to explore the behavioral and neural changes that occur with stimulation and treatment of clients in rehabilitation. We further need to know the expected duration and degree of generalizability of motor learning in relation to the training methods and learning structures we use. And, most importantly, we need to identify and measure the stimulus and reinforcement conditions that most reliably lead to the learning and retaining of therapeutic change. Such information will depend on cellular and whole animal physiologic and morphologic analysis of the events associated with the different paradigms of learning.

The issue of stimulus generalization (or transfer of training) is a critical dimension in the selection of therapeutic activity. Obviously, we are interested in developing total *patterns* of skill rather than *splinter* skills. To do this we need to know which qualities of stimulation and reinforcement (from therapeutic activities) lead to the quickest acquisition, longest retention, and most reliable transfer of skills from the learning environment to the person's own natural environment.

Consider the situation of the adult with postcerebrovascular accident (CVA) hemiplegia. If therapists use a neurodevelopmental approach to treating grasp-release deficits of the hand, they bias early relearning experiences toward the use of the ulnar types of grasp (i.e., hook, cylindrical, spherical) which tend to appear first developmentally in the acquisition of skilled hand use. Another statement of this bias would be to say that such an approach emphasizes power grip and the use of relatively large objects and tools. Whether such training then transfers any benefit to the radial hand functions (precision grasp and release of small objects with tip prehension and opposition patterns) depends on the degree to which there is generalization of learning from gross grasp and release tasks to fine grasp and release activities. Furthermore, such an approach assumes (without supporting empirical evidence) that generalization will be greater from gross to fine, ulnar to radial, than the reverse sequence. I am not attempting to argue the relative merits of developmental or recapitulation approaches verses other approaches. I wish to demonstrate that there may be unexplored, yet researchable issues concerning therapeutic learning that have never been explicitly examined. We would all prefer to know what the optimal mixture and optimal sequencing for such treatments should be. What is the optimal mixture of using small tools or no tools as opposed to only larger, heavier tools? What we cannot do with the present state of the art vis-a-vis therapeutic learning is reliably predict the consequences of one treatment approach and reinforcement schedule in comparison to other approaches. Until we investigate and understand the basic issues concerning the relationships of stimuli and reinforcers to motor learning and the nature and extent of stimulus generalization learning that is likely to occur, we are unable to answer the previous questions.

What kinds of variables should therapists be studying to answer these important issues? Clearly it needs to be established with clinical data that the proposed sequence of progression from short- to long-term learning paradigms is valid with respect to clinical situations. Physiologic studies using evoked cortical and brainstem potentials, electromyography, electrogoniometry, computerized ergometric tools, and other devices that can measure aggregate activity of small cellular systems (i.e., a single muscle) are needed to confirm that postulated temporal relationships between types of stimulation and the longevity of learning produced does indeed occur as predirected. Attempts to correlate human studies with those of lower species should be encouraged. Certainly we must look for the analogues of cellular events in the performance measures we use to assess therapeutic changes.

There is a need to evaluate currently used clinical methods to determine which of these represent PTP, PTD, habituation, sensitization, and classical and operant conditioning. The longer lasting learning approaches are relatively easy to identify, but it is not always so simple to determine whether facilitation/inhibition techniques are reflexive, PTP, PTD, or some combination of these.

Habituation procedures are certainly incorporated into a number of our treatment regimens but they have never been studied as such. Important questions include: Does overtraining have the predicted effect of increasing the longevity of habituation? Is serial habituation a viable approach to such syndromes as tactile defensiveness? What are optimal periods of stimulation? What are optimal frequencies of repetition of stimulation? To the extent that such techniques are presently reasonably effective, answers to these questions should maximize the benefits of these approaches.

The issues of massed versus distributed practice are also deserving of attention and research scrutiny. Obviously many clinicians let their practice schedules be dictated by the schedules of the setting in which they practice. Wherever treatment periods are scheduled to begin and end on the hour and/or half-hour or when patients cannot be seen more than once a day without having to be billed for multiple treatments, there are constraints on learning imposed by therapy *that are not necessarily in the best interests of either patient or therapist.* If we could document the influence of practice schedules on therapeutic outcomes, we might challenge successfully the administrative and customary rituals that limit our options in the design and execution of therapy.

Partial versus whole-task learning is another area that has not been adequately explored. Do we tend to use partial-task approaches with clients who have the cognitive ability to delay gratification and utilize conscious strategies during whole-task practice? Thousands of times I have witnessed therapists who were unable to stand by and permit the patient to practice an entire skill. Such therapists have an almost pathologic need to analyze performance into compartments and to stop patients whenever there are errors in performance and try to correct them immediately. This type of interference, albeit well intentioned, has led some therapists to be totally unable to ever permit true whole-task practice.

Whether forward or reverse chaining of responses is the preferred approach also requires further study. I am especially interested in whether there is a benefit to be realized by treating motor planning (praxic) deficit conditions with reverse chaining sequences. My own experiences with adults post-CVA having dyspraxic behavior has convinced me that there are certain benefits to reverse chaining with respect to the client's self-perceptions and self-evaluations, but I have no controlled or otherwise systematic data to suggest that this sequence is *more* appropriate than forward chaining. I subscribe to reverse chaining for the psychological value and reinforcement value, but need further evidence that this is indeed appropriate and not detrimental to the recovery of function.

As one who has used biofeedback for almost 10 years and has taught many others instrumentation, protocol design, hands-on skills, and treatment design, including the use of appropriate therapeutic learning activities, I am still not certain in many cases what are the relevant reinforcers and relevant eliciting stimuli for client behaviors.

Biofeedback, which has been relatively well documented as an adjunctive or supporting measure in therapy, has not been adequately investigated with respect to which stimuli and responses are the ones that lead to behavior changes. Studies of placebo effects in biofeedback suggest that the novelty of the equipment itself may heighten the arousal of learners. This may be a possible example of sensitization and should be investigated.

With respect to operant conditioning, useful studies would be those that seek to identify optimal reinforcement schedules for different conditions and different patients. Such information is well known and is critically dependent on individual variables such as motivation, arousal, attention, and previous history of rewards and punishments. What is needed is evidence that those therapists who consciously *apply* planned schedules of reinforcement fare better than those who only vaguely understand and/or apply such methods of operant conditioning.

The use of computer games, computer-assisted instruction (CAI), and computerized cognitive perceptual-motor evaluations and treatments is becoming increasingly widespread. This raises a number of important issues related to therapeutic learning. Do computerized evaluations and treatment enhance patient outcomes by rigorously controlling feedback? Is the computer a more effective means of feedback since it can be programmed to follow a defined reinforcement schedule? I believe that the absence of "punishment" in most forms of CAI leads to better extinction of undesirable behaviors and better retention of desirable activity. These and related issues concerning the relationship of learning theories to high technology intervention deserve further study.

In all areas of treatment and with each of the learning paradigms it will be interesting to see if evidence can be found to support the major thesis of this text: Therapists who understand and apply the principles of learning to their treatments will enhance their own effectiveness. A related issue that especially fascinates me is whether an understanding of learning principles will enable therapists to be more effective in analyzing and interpreting their own behaviors. I am of the opinion that many of the failures I have seen in my career as a therapist were my own failures to appreciate the situations in which I did not act to facilitate therapeutic learning and may have impeded such learning. Now that my interest in learning has led me to be more aware of my actions in learning situations, I have come to believe that "teaching disabilities" are a far more serious problem than "learning disabilities."

One other personal reflection on adopting the viewpoint that therapy is learning is that my attitude toward errors and mistakes, both my own and those of others, has changed dramatically. Such behaviors used to upset and arouse my emotions. I tended to interpret them as failure. I no longer do so. Mistakes and errors are part of our learning to generalize our responses. They are an essential part of the trial-and-error component of learning. If mistakes were never made there would be no awareness of the negative consequences, or at least the absence of reinforcement, of behaviors that are maladaptive. As a therapist I find that the analysis of errors is most important in developing methods of performance that avoid such errors on future trials. The only errors or mistakes that are problematic are those that are not recognized and not corrected.

By considering therapy as learning it becomes more pleasurable and more interesting. Every treatment should be designed not only to help the patient learn behaviors that will enable a more independent and dignified level of functioning, but also each treatment should be an opportunity to learn more about oneself and how we can improve our effectiveness. It is in this spirit of excitement and self-exploration that I have chosen to share this viewpoint with other clinicians. I hope it will prove useful to everyone who has explored this subject. I also hope that those who have been persistent and dedicated enough to read this book will never again be able to treat patients without thinking of therapy as learning.

References

Abildness AH: *Biofeedback Strategies*. Rockville, MD: American Occupational Therapy Association, 1982.

Ayres AJ: Occupational therapy for motor disorders resulting from impairment of the central nervous system. *J Rehab Lit* 21:202–310; 1970.

Ayres AJ: *Sensory Integration and Learning Disorders*. Los Angeles: Western Psychological Services, 1972.

Ayres AJ: *The Development of Sensory Integrative Theory and Practice*. Dubuque, IA: Kendall/Hunt Publishing, 1974.

Ayres AJ: *Interpreting the Southern California Sensory Integration Tests*. Los Angeles: Western Psychological Services, 1976.

Ayres AJ: *Sensory Integration and the Child*. Los Angeles: Western Psychological Services, 1980.

Bandura A: *Principles of Behavior Modification*. New York: Holt, Rinehart, and Winston, 1969.

Barr ML, Kiernan JA: *The Human Nervous System: An anatomical viewpoint*, 4th ed. Philadelphia: Harper & Row, 1983.

Beswick FB, Conroy, RTWL: Optimal tetanic conditioning of heteronymous monosynaptic reflexes. *J Physiol* 180:134–146; 1965.

Bishop B: Neurophysiology of motor responses evoked by vibratory stimulation. *Physical Ther* 54(12):1273–1282; 1974.

Bishop B: Possible applications of vibration in treatment of motor dysfunctions. *Physical Ther* 55(2):139–143; 1975.

Bishop PD, Kimmel HD: Retention of habituation and conditioning. *J Exp Psychol* 81(2):317–321; 1969.

Bitterman ME: The comparative analysis of learning: Are the laws of learning the same in all animals? *Science* 188(16):699–709; 1975.

Brady JV: Learning and conditioning. In *Behavioral Medicine: Theory and Practice*. OF Pomerleau, JP Brady, Editors. Baltimore: Williams and Wilkins, 1979.

Brake SC: Sucking infant rats learn a preference for a novel olfactory stimulus paired with milk delivery. *Science* 211:506–508, 1981.

Brodal A: *Neurological Anatomy in Relation to Clinical Medicine*, 3rd ed. New York: Oxford University Press, 1981.

Brons J, Woody CD: Long-term changes in excitability of cortical neurons after Pavlovian conditioning and extinction. *J Neurophysiol* 44:605–615; 1980.

Brunelli M, Castellucci V, Kandel ER: Synaptic facilitation and behavioral sensitization in aplysia: Possible role of scrotonin and cyclic AMP. *Science* 194:1178–1181; 1976.

Bruner J, Kennedy D: Habituation: Occurrence at a neuromuscular junction. *Science* 169:92–94; 1970.

Brunnstrom S: *Movement Therapy in Hemiplegia.* New York: Harper and Row, 1970.

Buchtel HA, Berlucci G: Learning, memory, and the nervous system. In *The Encyclopedia of Ignorance,* R Duncan, M Weston-Smith, Editors. Oxford, England: Pergamon Press, 1977.

Bullock TH: *Introduction to Nervous Systems.* San Francisco: W.H. Freeman and Co., 1977.

Burnside IG, Tobias HS, Bursill D: Electromyographic feedback in the remobilization of stroke patients: A controlled trial. *Arch Phys Med Rehabil* 63:217–222; 1982.

Carew TJ: Reflex action. In *Principles of Neural Science.* ER Kandel, JH Schwartz, Editors. New York: Elsevier, North-Holland, 1981.

Carew TJ, Walters ET, Kandel ER: Associative learning in aplysia: Cellular correlates supporting a conditioned fear hypothesis. *Science* 211:301–503; 1981.

Castellucci V, Kandel ER: Presynaptic facilitation as a mechanism for behavioral sensitization in aplysia. *Science* 194:1174–1178; 1976.

Cooper JR, Bloom FE, Roth RH: *The Biochemical Basis of Neuropharmacology,* 3rd ed. New York: Oxford University Press, 1978.

Cooper SS: Methods of teaching—Revisited games and simulation. *J Continuing Ed Nursing* H–J 14:47–48; 1979.

Cross KD: Role of practice in perceptual-motor learning. *Am J Phys Med* 46(1):487–510; 1967.

Crossman ERFW: Theory of acquisitions of speed-skill. *Ergonomics* 2:153–166; 1959.

Diamond S, Medina J, Diamond-Falk J, DeVeno T: The value of biofeedback in the treatment of chronic headache: A five-year retrospective study. *Headache* 19(2):90–96; 1979.

Douglas WW: Stimulus-secretion coupling: The concept and clues from chromaffin and other cells. *Br J Pharmacol* 34:451–474; 1968.

Dudel J, Kuffler SW: Presynaptic inhibition at the crayfish neuromuscular junction. *J Physiol* (Lond) 155:543–562; 1961.

Eccles JC: The neurophysiological basis of mind. *The Principles of Neurophysiology.* Oxford, England: Clarendon Press, 1953.

Eccles JC: *The Physiology of Synapses.* Berlin: Springer, 1964.

Ethridge D: Commentary on Smith and Tempone. *Am J Occup Ther* 22:420–422; 1968.

Evans B: Learned responses to movement in neonates. *Dev Psychobiol* 13:95–110; 1980.

Evarts EV, Hughes JR: Relationship of posttetanic potentiation to subnormality of lateral geniculate potentials. *Am J Physiol* 188:238–244; 1957.

Farber SD: *Neurorehabilitation: A Multisensory Approach.* Philadelphia: W.B. Saunders, 1982.

Feuerstein R: Ontogeny of learning in man. In *Brain Mechanisms in Memory and Learning: From the Single Neuron to Man.* MAB Brazier, Editor. *Int Brain Res Org Monogr* Series, No. 4. New York: Raven Press, 1979, pp. 361–372.

Fiorentini A, Berardi N: Perceptual learning specific for orientation and spatial frequency. *Nature* 287:43–44; 1980.

Fiorentini M: *Reflex Testing Methods for Evaluating Central Nervous System Development*, 2nd ed. Springfield, IL: Charles C. Thomas, 1973.

Fisher AG, Dunn W: Tactile defensiveness: Historical perspectives, new research—A theory grows. *Sensory Integration Special Interest Section Newsletter*, AOTA, 6(2):1–2; 1983.

Foreman J, Mongar J: Calcium and the control of histamine secretion from mast cells. In *Calcium Transport in Contraction and Secretion.* E Carafoli, F Clementi, W Drabikowski, A Margerth, Editors. New York: American Elsevier, 1975.

Freud S: *An Outline of Psychoanalysis*, Trans. 1949. New York: Norton and Co., 1940.

Gatchel RJ, Price KP: *Clinical Applications for Biofeedback: Appraisal and Status.* New York: Pergamon Press, 1979.

Gillies D, Lance JW, Neilson PD, et al.: Presynaptic inhibition of the monosynaptic reflex by vibration. *J Physiol* 205:329–339; 1969.

Ginott HG: *Between Parent & Child.* New York: Macmillan Co., 1965.

Gissen AJ, Katz RL: Twitch, tetanus and post-tetanic potentiation as indices of nerve-muscle block in man. *J Anesthesiol* 30:5; 1969.

Granit R: *The Purposive Brain.* Cambridge, MA: MIT Press, 1977.

Greenbaum H: The learning process in combined psychotherapy. *Am J Psychoanal* 39(4):303–310; 1979.

Harris FA: Multiple-loop modulation of motor outflow. *Phys Ther* 51(4):391–397; 1971.

Harris FA, Spelman FA, Hymer JW: Electronic sensory aids as treatment for cerebral-palsied children. *Phys Ther* 54(4):354–365; 1974.

Hayes KC, Clarke AM: Learning effect in human muscular responses to proprioceptive stimuli. *Physiol Behav* 21:57–63; 1978.

Hearst E: The classical-instrumental distinction: Reflexes, voluntary behavior and the categories of associative learning. In *Handbook of Learning and Cognitive Processes, Vol. 2, Conditioning and Behavior Therapy.* WK Estes, Editor. Hillsdale, NJ: Lawrence Erlbaum Associate, 1975.

Hollis LI: Skinnerian occupational therapy. *Am J Occup Ther* 28(4):208–213; 1974.

Holt G: Patient characteristics: How adults learn. *Am Pharm* NS21 (7):46–47, 70, 1981.

Hull CL: Stimulus intensity dynamism (v) and stimulus generalizations. *Psychol Rev* 36(2):67–76; 1940.

Hunt WA, Matarazzo JD, Weiss SM, Gentry WD: Associative learning, habit, and health behavior. *J Behav Med* 2(2):111–124; 1979.

Hutter OF: Post-tetanic restoration of neuromuscular transmission blocked by D-tubocurarine. *J Physiol* 118:216; 1952.

Iverson LL: The chemistry of the brain. *The Brain.* San Francisco: W.H. Freeman and Co., 1979.

Jeffrey WE: The orienting reflex and attention in cognitive development. *Psychol Rev* 75:320–334; 1968.

Kandel ER: Calcium and the control of synaptic strength by learning. *Nature* 293:697–700; 1981.

Kandel ER: A cell-biological approach to learning. *Grass lecture Monogr 1.* Bethesda, MD: Society for Neuroscience, 1979a.

Kandel ER: Psychotherapy and the single synapse: The impact of psychiatric thought on neurobiologic research. *N Engl J Med* 301(19):1028–1037; 1979b.

Kandel ER: Cellular aspects of learning. In *Brain Mechanisms in Memory and Learning from the Single Neuron to Man.* M Brazier, Editor. New York: Raven Press, 1979c.

Kandel ER: Cellular insights into behavior and learning. *Harvey Lecture Ser* 73:19–92; 1979d.

Kandel ER: *Cellular Basis of Behavior: An Introduction to Behavioral Neurobiology.* San Francisco: W.H. Freeman and Co., 1976.

Katz B: *The Release of Neural Transmitter Substances.* Springfield, IL: Charles C. Thomas, 1969.

Katz B, Miledi R: The effect of calcium on acetylcholine release from motor nerve terminals. *Proc R Soc Lond* (Biol) 161:496–503; 1965.

Kennedy R: The Rubro Olivo-cerebellar teaching circuit. *Med Hypotheses* 5:799–807; 1979.

Konorski J: *Conditioned Reflexes and Neuron Organization.* England: Cambridge University Press, reprinted 1968.

Kottke FJ: From reflex to skill: The training of coordination. *Arch Phys Med Rehabil* 61:551–561; 1980.

Krussen FH, Kottke FJ, Ellwood PM: *Handbook of Physical Medicine and Rehabilitation,* 2nd ed. Philadelphia: WB Saunders Company, 1971.

Kuffler SW, Edwards C: Mechanism of gamma aminobutyric acid (GABA) action and its relation to synaptic inhibition. *J Neurophysiol* 21:589–610; 1958.

Kupferman I: Neurophysiology of learning. *Annu Rev Psychol* 26:367–391; 1975.

Kupferman I: Learning. In *Principles of Neuralscience.* ER Kandel, JH Schwartz, Editors. New York: Elsevier, North-Holland, Inc., 1981.

Kushner HS: *When Bad Things Happen to Good People.* New York: Schocken Books, 1981.

Larrabee MG, Bronk DW: Prolonged facilitation of synaptic excitability in sympathetic ganglia. *J Neurophysiol* 10:139–159; 1947.

Lee C, Barnes A, Yang E, Katy RL: Neuromuscular facilitation during train-of-four and tetanic stimulation in healthy volunteers: Observations with half-refractory paired responses. *Br. J. Anaesth* 49:555; 1977.

Liley AW: The quantal components of the mammalian end-plate potential. *J Physiol* (Lond) 133:571–587; 1956.

Lloyd DPC: Post-tetanic potentiation of response in monosynaptic reflex pathways of the spinal cord. *J Gen Physiol* 33:147–170; 1949.

Logue AW: Taste aversion and the generality of the laws of learning. *Psychol Bull* 86(2):276–296; 1979.

Lucca JA, Recchiuti SJ: Effect of electromyographic biofeedback or an isometric strengthening program. *Phys Ther* 63(2):200–203; 1983.

Martin I, Levey AB: *The Genesis of the Classically Conditioned Response.* Oxford, England: Pergamon Press Ltd., 1969.

Matsumura M, Woody CD: Excitability increases in facial motoneurons of the cat after serial presentations of glabella tap. Bethesda, MD: *Soc Neuroscience Abstr* 6:78; 1980.

Moore JC: Neuroanatomical consideration relating to recovery of function following brain lesions. In *Recovery of Function: Theoretical Considerations for Brain Injury Rehabilitation.* P Bach-y-Rita, Editor. Baltimore: University Park Press, 1980.

Mpitsos GJ, Collins SD, McClellan AD: Learning: A model system for physiological studies. *Science* 199:497–506; 1978.

Munsinger H: *Fundamentals of Child Development.* New York: Holt, Rinehart, and Winston, Inc., 1975.

Murphy RJ, Doughty NR: Establishment of controlled arm movements in profoundly retarded students using response contingent vibratory stimulation. *Am J Ment Defic* 82(2):212–216; 1977.

Noback CR, Demarest RJ: *The Human Nervous System: Basic Principles of Neurobiology,* 2nd ed. New York: McGraw-Hill Book Company, 1975.

Norman CW: Behavior modification: A perspective. *Am J Occup Ther* 30(8):491–497; 1967.

Pavlov IP: The scientific investigation of the psychical faculties of processes in higher animals. *Science* 24:613–619; 1906.

Peck JB: Commentary on Smith and Tempone. *Am J Occup Ther* 22:423–425; 1968.

Petrinovich L, Patterson TL: Field studies of habituation: I. Effect of reproductive condition, number of trials, and different delay intervals on responses of the white-crowned sparrow. *J Comp Physiol Psych* 93(2):337–350; 1979.

Pomerleau OF, Brady JP, Editors. *Behavioral Medicine Theory and Practice.* Baltimore: Williams and Wilkins, 1979.

Rasch PJ, Burke RK: *Kinesiology and Applied Anatomy.* Philadelphia: Lea and Febiger, 1974.

Reeve TG, Magill RA: The role of the components of knowledge of results information in error correction. *Res Q Exerc Sport* 52(1):80–85; 1981.

Rogers C: *Freedom to Learn.* Columbus, OH: Charles E. Merrill Publishing Company, 1969.

Rovetto F: Treatment of chronic constipation by classical conditioning techniques. *J Behav Ther Exp Psychiat* 10:143–146; 1979.

Scholz J, Campbell S: Muscle spindles and the regulation of movement. *Phys Ther* 60(11):1416–1424; 1980.

Schwartz GE, Shapiro D, Tursky B: Learned control of cardiovascular integration in man through operant conditioning. *Psychosom Med* 33:57–62; 1971.

Schwartz RK: Olfaction and muscle activity: An EMG pilot study. *Am J Occup Ther* 33:185–192; 1979.

Schwartz RK: Therapy as learning. Paper presented at the 1980 AOTA annual conference, Denver, 1980.

Seligman MEP: On the generality of the laws of learning. *Psychol Rev* 77:406–418; 1970.

Shaperman J: Learning patterns of young children with above-elbow prostheses. *Am J Occup Ther* 33(5):299–305; 1979.

Singer R, Pease D: Effect of guided versus discovery learning strategies on initial motor task learning, transfer and retention. *Res Q* 49(2):206–217; 1978.

Singer SJ, Nicolson GL: The fluid mosaic model of the structure of cell membranes. *Science* 175:720; 1972.

Skinner BF: *The Behavior of Organisms.* New York: Appleton-Century-Crofts, 1938.

Skinner BF: *Science and Human Behavior.* New York: The Free Press, 1965.

Solomonow M, Herskovitz JS, Lyman J: Learning in the tactile sense. *Ann Biomed Engin* 7:127–134; 1979.

Stein F: A current review of the behavioral frame of reference and its application to occupational therapy. In *Psychiatric Occupational Therapy: A Holistic Approach.* F Stein, Editor. Philadelphia: F.A. Davis, 1983.

Stern D: Play and learning in the first year: New insights. *Pediatr Nursing Suppl* B-6:55; 1979.

Stockmeyer S: An interpretation of the approach of Rood to the treatment of neuromuscular dysfunction. *Am J Phys Med* 46(1):900–956; 1967.

Thompson RF, Spencer WA: Habituation: A model phenomenon for the study of neuronal substrates of behavior. *Psychol Rev* 73(1):16–43; 1966.

Thorndike EL: Animal intelligence—An experimental study of associative processes in animals. *Psychol Monog Suppl* No. 8: 1–106, 1898.

Thorpe WH: *Learning and Instruction in Animals.* London: Methuen 1956, p.54.

Trombly CA: Principles of operant conditioning: Related to orthotic training of quadriplegic patients. *Am J Occup Ther* 20(5):217–220; 1966.

Trombly CA: *Occupational Therapy for Physical Dysfunction,* 2nd ed. Baltimore: Williams and Wilkins, 1983.

Wall PD: Habituation and post-tetanic potentiation in the spinal cord. In *Short-term Changes in Neural Activity and Behavior.* G Horn, RA Hinde, Editors. New York: Cambridge University Press, 1970.

Wallace SA, Hagler RW: Knowledge of performance and the learning of a closed motor skill. *Res Q* 50(2):265–271; 1979.

Walters ET, Carew TJ, Kande ER: Classical conditioning in aplysia Californica. *Proc Natl Acad Sci USA* 76(12):6675–6679; 1979.

Waziri R, Kandel ER, Frazier WT: Organization of inhibition in abdominal ganglion of aplysia. II. Posttetanic frequency of inhibitory post synaptic potentials. *J Neurophysiol* V32:509–519; 1969.

White RR: Motivation reconsidered: The concept of competence. *Psychol Rev* 56:297–333; 1959.

Woody CD: *Memory, Learning, and Higher Function: A Cellular View.* New York: Springer-Verlag, 1982.

Yu J: Neuromuscular recovery with training after central nervous system lesions: An experimental approach. Personal Correspondence.

Glossary

Absolute refractory period: The time period following the generation of an action potential during which the neuron is incapable of responding to a stimulus no matter how great the stimulus strength.

Action potential: Time-dependent, all-or-none, fixed amplitude (nondecremental), self-propagating series of electrical waves of activity (polarizations and depolarizations) transmitted across the cell membranes of neurons during the transmission of a nerve impulse and/or across the cell membranes of muscle cells during excitation and contraction of the muscle cell.

Adaptation: The decline in generator potential amplitude (and hence, decrease in frequency of action potentials) in afferent neurons in response to continuous stimulation at a fixed or constant intensity.

Afferent: Moving from the periphery toward the central nervous system, especially with reference to the transmission of sensory action potentials from peripheral receptors toward more central and/or rostral central nervous system structures.

Afterdischarge: An integrative phenomenon whereby divergent postsynaptic action potentials lead to continued action potential activity which outlasts the stimulus leading to primary action potentials in sensory neurons.

Appetitive conditioning: Learning that occurs as a result of providing a positive reward or pleasurable stimulus; this is specifically used in classical conditioning to refer to the association of a pleasurable or rewarding unconditional stimulus with a conditional stimulus to result in consummatory or approach behavior as the conditioned response.

Association neurons: Nerve cells that are neither motor nor sensory with respect to their function; instead they serve to exchange, process, and integrate information within the nervous system region in which they are located. Association neurons tend to be Golgi type II (local circuitry) neurons.

Associative learning: Learning that occurs as the direct result of the close temporal pairing of stimuli as with the conditioned stimulus and unconditioned stimulus in classical conditioning.

127

Autogenic training: Self-produced or self-mediated learning in which one produces mental images or intrinsic stimuli to elicit or alter specific physiologic responses.

Aversive conditioning: Learning in which painful or unpleasant stimuli are used to suppress or eliminate undesirable behaviors.

Behavior modification: The systematic application of learning theories to alter the observable behaviors of clients via the controlled use of stimuli to habituate, sensitize, or classically or operantly condition responses.

Biofeedback: The detection, amplification, and display of physiologic events such as electrical activity of muscle, skin temperature, heart rate, etc., so that with this information the individual can control and alter behavior; also refers to a systematic approach to therapy, using information concerning the client's own physiologic responses to teach that person to control responses.

Capacitance: The ability to store and separate electric charges when two conducting elements are separated by a non-conducting element.

Classical conditioning: The learning process whereby the repeated pairing of an ineffective or neutral stimulus with a stimulus that invariably elicits a response eventually results in the development of the ability of the neutral stimulus alone to elicit the response (or one that closely resembles it).

Competence drives: Persistent tendencies of individual animals or persons to explore, manipulate, and move within an environmental context and thereby develop abilities and skills to enable them to survive and reproduce.

Compound schedule of reinforcement: A set of rules requiring the criteria of two or more schedules of reinforcement be met before reinforcement is provided.

Concurrent schedule of reinforcement: A set of rules permitting reinforcement to be given only if two or more behaviors (operants) meet the simultaneous demands of two or more reinforcement schedules.

Conditioned (or conditional) stimulus: Any neutral stimulus incapable of eliciting a specific response unless it is repeatedly paired with a stimulus that invariably elicits that response.

Continuous reinforcement: A set of rules for providing reinforcement, which requires that every operant response be reinforced.

Convergence: The integrative mechanism whereby two or more neurons synapse upon a single postsynaptic neuron.

Defensive conditioning: The form of learning in which noxious or punitive stimuli are used to establish behaviors which are protective in nature and/or to establish behaviors which tend to escape or avoid such stimuli.

Depolarization: A decrease in electrical polarity, usually produced by an increase in the permeability of the nerve or muscle cell membrane to sodium ions.

Dishabituation: A form of sensitization characterized by the use of a sudden novel or strong stimulus to restore the original amplitude (strength) of a habituated response.

Distributed practice: The practice of following each learning trial with a period of rest before beginning another learning trial.

Divergence: The integrative mechanism whereby a single neuron synapses upon two or more postsynaptic neurons.

Efferent: Moving from the central nervous system toward the periphery, especially with reference to the flow of action potentials to effector organs such as glands and muscles; used often to refer to "motor" pathways of the nervous system.

Electromotive force: The ability of voltage or potential of unlike charges separated by some distance to do work.

Encoded: Translate information or stimulus energy into a simplified form, such as patterns of action potentials within the nervous system.

End plate potential (EPP): The depolarization that results from the release of acetylcholine and its action at the postsynaptic membrane of the neuromuscular junction.

Equilibrium potential: The membrane potential for a given ion at which there is no net movement of an ion across a semipermeable membrane because the force of ionic concentration gradients is equal and opposite to the electromotive potential difference across the membranes.

Excitatory postsynaptic potential (EPSP): A graded depolarization of a postsynaptic neuron produced by the release of an "excitatory" neurotransmitter and generally due to an increase in postsynaptic membrane permeability to all small ions.

Extinction: A procedure for eliminating conditioned responses, e.g., the repeated presentation of conditioned stimulus not followed by presentation of unconditioned stimulus in classical conditioning which decreases the likelihood of conditioned response to presentation of conditioned stimulus.

Facilitation: In a general sense this is the enhancement or reinforcement of a behavior, which allows it to be carried out with greater ease; in a specific sense it refers to a lowering of the action potential threshold of a neuron in response to prior activity of that neuron (as with post-tetanic potentiation).

Fluid mosaic model (of Singer): A dynamic model of the cell membrane in which membrane proteins are characterized as "floating" in a fluid, phospholipid bilayer.

Forward chaining: An approach in which the component acts of a given task are learned in their natural order of appearance, i.e., those actions performed first are learned first and subsequent actions of a given sequence are only learned when all prior steps have been learned.

Frequency coded: Information that is conveyed by the numbers of action potentials per unit time as, for example, the coding of stimulus intensity by many afferent neurons so that the greater the stimulus strength, the higher the resulting frequencies of action potentials in the primary afferent neurons.

Ganglia: Any collection of neuronal cell bodies that lies outside of the central nervous system.

Generator potential: A graded (decremental), stimulus-induced change in the membrane potential of a sensory receptor which can initiate action potentials in sensory neurons by depolarizing the membrane adjacent to the sensory receptor to its threshold level.

Graded potentials: Variable amplitude depolarizations and hyperpolarizations of neuronal membranes most often seen at sensory receptors and postsynaptic nerve and myoneural junctions. These are in distinct contrast to action potentials that are *fixed* amplitude responses of neurons to suprathreshold depolarizations.

Habituation: A reversible decrease in the amplitude (strength) of a response when it is repeatedly elicited using non-noxious stimulation.

Heterosynaptic: Characterizes a process in which activity in a stimulated or activated afferent pathway can alter the responses of a neuron to other non-stimulated pathways.

Homosynaptic: Characterizes a process in which responses to stimulation change as a result of activity in a single afferent pathway but remain unchanged in response to activity in other afferent pathways.

Hyperpolarization: An increase in electrical polarity across a nerve or muscle cell membrane which tends to move the membrane potential further away from the action potential threshold.

Inhibition: Any process which reduces or stops a behavior; in a more specific sense it refers to those neural events that decrease the likelihood of action potentials occurring in a given neuron or muscle cell.

Inhibitory postsynaptic potentials (IPSP): A graded hyperpolarization of a postsynaptic neuron produced by the release of an "inhibitory" neurotransmitter and generally due to an increase in membrane permeability to chloride ions.

Instrumental conditioning (also known as operant conditioning): The presentation of a reinforcing stimulus after the occurrence of a given response so that repeated presentations of the reinforcing stimulus lead to an increase in the frequency and/or probability of the reinforced response.

Integration: Those mechanisms or processes whereby the output signals of single cells or assemblies of cells are determined as a function of their input signals.

Interval reinforcement: Reinforcement at specified time intervals during performance, independent of how many times the operant behavior has occurred.

Knowledge of results: A conscious evaluation of the degree of success (and/or failure) of an action after its completion; also used to refer to such an assessment with respect to its value as feedback to be used to modify subsequent behaviors.

Learning: The process whereby an individual modifies responsiveness to stimuli or acquires new patterns of behavior as a result of previous interactions with the environment, not including those changes due to growth, maturation, or aging, those caused by disease or trauma, or those that reflect a change in levels of awareness or motivation.

Length constant: The distance over which a voltage applied to a membrane decays to approximately one-third of its original value. This varies from neuron to neuron and even within regions of the membrane of a single neuron.

Masking of recovery: The phenomenon in which secondary deficits, not part of a primary pathologic condition, limit or obscure the functional expression of resolution or recovery from primary symptoms. For example, biomechanical limitations such as disuse atrophy or contractures may lead to a false impression that nervous system paralysis limits the client's ability to move even when neural recovery is extensive or even complete.

Massed practice: The repetition of a learning trial without any period of rest between one learning trial and the next.

Mediated learning experience: A situation in which the learning individual is assisted by another person whose role is to organize, interpret, and force relevant stimuli on the learner.

Miniature end plate potential (MEPP): The small spontaneous depolarizations of muscle cells which are thought to be the result of the random leakage of the contents of a single or several presynaptic vesicles of neurotransmitter at the myoneural junction.

Motor unit: Used to describe an individual alpha motor neuron and all of the muscle fibers that it innervates.

Multiple schedule of reinforcement: Rules that require complex conditions, not easily classified under commonly used categories of reinforcement schedules, to be met as a condition for the provision of reinforcement.

Myelin: The substance that constitutes the axonal sheaths of many neurons. The highly lipid or fat content gives a characteristic white appearance to such axons. Myelin is formed by the membrane laminations of Schwann cells in the peripheral nervous system and membrane laminations of oligodendroglia cells within the central nervous system.

Negative reinforcement: Any situation in which the termination of a stimulus increases the probability of an operant response.

Neurotransmitter: A chemical substance stored and released by neurons into the synaptic cleft that subsequently reacts with specialized receptor sites on the postsynaptic cell to produce changes in membrane permeability.

Nuclei: A collection or aggregation of nerve cell bodies within the central nervous system. Neurons of a given nuclei usually have structural and functional similarities to one another.

Operant conditioning: Another term for instrumental conditioning defined above.

Partial reinforcement schedules: Rules that provide only certain occasions of operant responding will be followed by reinforcement.

Partial task practice: A training or instructional approach which divides tasks into a series of components and requires that these components be learned to set criterion before the task is attempted as a complete and continuous action.

Perception: The organization and interpretation of sensory information by the nervous system.

Phasic receptors: Sensory receptor endings that have rapid adaptation to continuous stimulation.

Plasticity: Changes within neural systems that result in prolonged alteration of cellular and/or synaptic function which, in principle, could account for changes in behavior.

Place coded: Information conveyed by the anatomic location of neurons that receive information of a specific type from a given region of the body or given region of the nervous system.

Positive reinforcement: Any situation in which the presentation of a stimulus increases the probability of an operant response.

Post-tetanic depression: Repetitive, high-frequency stimulation of a neural pathway or muscle cell that results in a decrease in neuronal or muscle cell response to a stimulus as compared to responses to that same stimulus seen before tetanization.

Post-tetanic potentiation: Repetitive, high-frequency stimulation of a neural pathway or muscle cell that results in an increase in neuronal or muscle cell response to a stimulus as compared to responses to that same stimulus seen before tetanization.

Practice: The repetition of an act one or more times performed with the express goal of improving the learner's temporal and/or spatial control of that act.

Primary drive: The existence of a tissue deficit which motivates an organism to respond with certain species' characteristic behavior patterns.

Punishment: A noxious stimulus used to suppress or prevent the occurrence of a behavior.

Quantum unit of neurotransmitter: The smallest amount of neurotransmitter that can be released under natural conditions and which is generally accepted to be equivalent to the contents of a single presynaptic vesicle of neurotransmitter.

Ratio reinforcement schedule: Rules that stipulate how many times an operant behavior must occur before it is reinforced.

Rebound: A clinical situation in which a desirable therapeutic change in behavior is followed by a reversal of effect so that undesirable changes in behavior follow the desirable ones.

Reflex: A highly stereotyped, obligatory response to a particular stimulus in which the intensity of the response varies as a function of stimulus intensity.

Reinforcement: Any stimulus that alters the probability of a given response (operant) occurring.

Relative refractory period: A time during the repolarization of a neuron or muscle cell after an action potential, during which a suprathreshold stimulus may elicit another action potential even though the resting membrane potential of the cell has not yet been restored.

Resistance: That property of any material which restricts the flow of electrical charges and/or electrically charged particles.

Resistance to extinction: The degree to which an operantly conditioned behavior is maintained even when no reinforcement is provided.

Response generalization: The phenomenon in which a single habituation, sensitization, operant, or instrumental stimulus may be effective, with responses resembling the training response but more appropriate to the learner's environment.

Respondents: Behaviors or responses that are clearly evoked by an antecedent stimulus, such as reflex responses.

Resting membrane potential: Electrical potential difference between the inside of a cell and its surrounding extracellular environment. These do not vary from hour to hour but are constant. This potential is usually negative inside the cell with respect to outside the cell.

Reverse chaining: An approach in which the component acts of a given task are learned in the exact opposite of their natural sequence of occurrence.

Schedule of reinforcement: Criteria or rules that state under which circumstances specifically defined reinforcement will be provided.

Secondary drive: The tendency to respond with behaviors that lead to desirable or pleasurable consequences in the absence of tissue deficits. Such drives include the desire for recognition or approval and for money and material goods not essential to survival.

Sensitization: An increase in the amplitude (strength) of a response to a given stimulus as a result of the presentation of another stimulus, often very strong or noxious, where such enhancement does not depend on pairing of the stimuli.

Shaping (also known as training or learning by successive approximations): This consists of reinforcing in succession those responses that lead to the individual performing behaviors that over time come closer and closer to the desired result of such learning.

Spatial summation: The phenomenon of two or more postsynaptic potentials produced at the same point in time, but at different points on the nerve membrane, interacting to produce an integrated postsynaptic potential.

Stimulus generalization: The phenomenon in which stimuli similar to those used in training are used to elicit learned responses, reinforce voluntary responses, or fail to elicit habituated responses.

Synapse: The region of contact between neurons or between neurons and effector cells across which nervous impulses are transmitted chemically or electrically. At every synapse there exists potential for change in the postsynaptic cell's activity.

Synaptic vesicles: Membrane enclosed subcellular structures containing neurotransmitter found in presynaptic nerve terminals. These release their contents into the synaptic cleft via exocytosis.

Temporal summation: The phenomenon of two or more postsynaptic potentials produced at the same point on the neuronal membrane but at different points in time interacting to produce an integrated postsynaptic potential.

Threshold potential: The membrane potential at which an all-or-none action potential response occurs.

Time constant: The time over which a voltage applied to a membrane uses approximately two-thirds of its final value.

Transduced: To be changed from physical energy into some other form of activity (usually generator potentials) in sensory receptors.

Unconditional or unconditioned stimulus: Any stimulus that always elicits a predictable, stereotyped response.

Voltage: A measure of the potential of electrical charges separated by some distance to do work.

Voluntary response: One which is under the control of the will of the performer and unconstrained by obligatory stimulus-response relationships.

Whole-task practice: The repetition of a skill in its entirety, from beginning to end, over and over until the learning goal is reached.

Index